SARAH KEY'S
BACK SUFFERERS' BIBLE

SARAH KEY'S
Back Sufferers' Bible

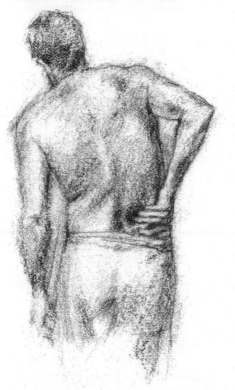

Allen & Unwin

First published in 2000

Allen & Unwin
9 Atchison Street
St Leonards NSW 2065
Australia
Phone: (61 2) 8425 0100
Fax: (61 2) 9906 2218
Email: frontdesk@allen-unwin.com.au
Web: http://www.allen-unwin.com.au

National Library of Australia
Cataloguing-in-Publication entry:

Key, Sarah.
Sarah Key's back sufferers' bible.

Bibliography.
Includes index.
ISBN 1 86508 321 6.

1. Back exercises. 2. Backache – Exercise therapy. 3. Backache – Treatment.
4. Spine – Instability – Exercise therapy. 5. Spine – Instability – Treatment. I. Title.

617.5606

Anatomical drawings: Philip Wilson
Figure illustrations: Robert Harvey
Index: Russell Brooks

Set in 11/14 pt Berkeley by Samphire Publishing Partners
Printed by Griffin Press, South Australia

10 9 8 7 6 5 4 3 2 1

Foreword

by HRH The Prince of Wales

ST. JAMES'S PALACE

Anyone writing about anything complicated knows how hard it is to hit the right note; to convey the right amount of information without lapsing into technical jargon so you leave your reading public behind and, at the same time, not dumbing it all down.

In this new book Sarah Key proposes, in readable language, a new framework for the way healthy spines break down through different stages and become painful. In a classic case of not seeing the wood for the trees, she believes that most spinal problems start off as a simple stiff link in the spine but it is so low-tech it escapes the attention of conventional medical 'wisdom'. Despite backpain being universally commonplace, she says it is often ignored until something more serious develops (like arthritis of the spine or a slipped disc) which is more easily recognised and diagnosed.

I find Sarah Key's book makes sense in what to many is a pretty incomprehensible subject. It is such a help to have it explained so one can actually understand what is going on. Visualising what is happening inside the back makes it much more logical and easy to see why Sarah Key's exercises really do work. After all, I should know. As one of her guinea pigs over the years I can vouch for their effectiveness, if not claim some credit for honing the final product.

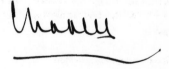

Contents

Acknowledgments

My thanks go to Nikolai Bogduk and Lance Twomey who wrote *my* bible *Clinical Anatomy of the Lumbar Spine* (Churchill Livingstone) and Anne Kern, my editor, who kept the faith when it was wearing thin.

Disclaimer

Your own physical condition and diagnosis may require specific modifications or precautions. Before undertaking any course of self treatment you should consult your doctor or health care provider.

To my husband and three children: Silkyskin, Milkyskin and Butterbody

Introduction

THE WAY IT MIGHT BE...

There is something sublimely beautiful in the way the human body moves which is often played out in sport. Something about the hum-drum splendour of each 'grand action', like a workaday form of ballet: the golfer leaning sideways into his swing and then winding up to the finish, his trunk twirled and elbows held high. Or the swimmer carving a furrow through the water, his body rolling languidly behind as his legs make their slow-motion, thin scissors kick.

I wonder too, whether some sporting actions affect us because they strike a deeper chord, echoing some long past function in our primitive memory; actions half forgotten, half innate. The spread-eagled star shape of the javelin thrower, at the point of letting it fly. Or the horse and its rider, both flattened out at the gallop, or better still the curling bursting thrust of a spine unravelling backwards, as the rower pulls his scull across the water.

To me, rowing is the most beautiful sporting action of all. And smitten as I am, I wonder if the instinct has been in my blood all along; some tenuous calling like a wispy, elusive thread through history, linking me to an earlier image of sunlight flashing on a flank of oars. Perhaps this fleeting resonance with the days of Phoenician galleys and Viking longboats has caused me—nearing the end of my fourth decade—to embark on my own odyssey by learning to row.

In that semi-transcendent state of synchronised exertion, as my white gloved hands describe neat semi-circles in to my ribs and I hear the muted clonk of the riggers as all eight blades turn and feather in unison, I feel I am in touch with something deeper than the mere thrill of bubbles bursting against the hull and the sun peeping over the headland, its first rays dancing in shards on the dimpled water.

With sweat trickling down my brow, in awe I watch the back of my crew-mate in front of me—because you never see a back working better than that. As she curls forward, hands stretched over the gunwales, legs loaded up at the catch, she is about to roll back in one beautifully timed flowing action where the power of her legs and trunk straightening, as her arms finish the stroke, adds up to a sum of energy greater than its parts.

For someone who has spent the whole of her professional life watching spines that can barely bend forward to pick up the toothpaste, I sense another confluence on why it is that things come to pass.

THE WAY IT IS...

Backpain is on the increase. There is probably not a soul on Earth who has not been troubled at some stage by it, or not known someone else who has. Because of our lifestyle, backpain is more widespread now than ever before. Universal automation has caused us to go soft and our spines struggle to cope with long periods of indolence punctuated by jarring over-exertion.

I suspect the origins of backpain are simpler than we ever dreamt possible: a benign 'linkage' problem caused by the stiffening of a disc-vertebra union at the front of the spine. As the disc dries and gets harder and the vertebra on top loses mobility, the segment becomes sluggish, like a stiff link in a bicycle chain. This is then the derivative spinal condition, and furthermore the starting point from which other more serious problems can flow.

All of us walking around have spines riddled with stiff links such as these, and never know they are there. They just lie there like sleepers and rarely come to light. But in some cases, and particularly in the lower spine which carries more weight, the link can become so stiff it becomes painful—and this, I believe, is the chief cause of common or garden backache.

People who use their hands to alleviate backache—such as physiotherapists, chiropractors, osteopaths and to some extent masseurs—can feel a painfully jammed segment, like a plug of cement in a rubber hose. Probing about with the thumbs or heel of the hand we can feel if a vertebra does not yield or is out of alignment; if it doesn't go it doesn't go.

Conventional orthopaedics has never recognised segmental stiffness as a subliminal spinal disorder—far less felt about for it with the hands—which makes it abundantly clear why our two strands of medicine to this day remain so divergent. For manual practitioners, who interface with the back-suffering public in droves, the concept is central to our thinking. Yet it still has no place in mainstream diagnostics. What we work on all the time has no name in the swathes of medical literature. I suspect it is too low tech; too simple for words.

I believe the medical profession has focused too deeply on backs, looking for cold hard 'evidence' instead of searching for something more subtle and reversible. Doctors tend to look for things which are lacking, or out of place, and which at worst they might remove. They seem fixated on taking pictures and doing tests, instead of keeping it simple (certainly in the first instance) by watching and feeling, like a piano tuner, for what the trouble might be.

By being too analytical they highlight complicated, unlikely causes of backpain—when all along, it may be some passing function fault in need of being handled right. And if cold hard evidence is lacking, another quandary can arise: the sufferer is disbelieved or worse still, dismissed as a malingerer.

Without using the hands, segmental stiffness is impossible to pick up. It never shows up with conventional imaging of X-rays and CT scans, any more than a photograph shows up a stiff hinge in a door. Recently however, developments have been more promising: highly accurate magnetic resonance imaging (MRI) is providing the first glimmer of evidence to corroborate what people like me can feel with our hands. With the quality improving all the time, perhaps before long MRI will 'see' the lowered water content in the tissues (from which it takes its signal) as the stiffness we manual operators can feel.

The fact remains: backpain is pandemic. It permeates all nationalities, all social groups and all professions, and in modern times is second only to the common cold as a cause of time off work. There are literally millions upon millions of sufferers in the world today no closer to having their questions answered or their problem solved. A recent survey carried out in Britain discovered 'a profound and widespread dissatisfaction with what is at present available to help people who suffer from back pain' (Department of Health and Social Security, 1996). Likewise, in the United States 85 per cent of the people who visit their medical practitioner 'leave with no nuts and bolts reason for their pain' (*Scientific American*, August 1998). At the beginning of the new millennium it seems we are little further ahead. In a manner of speaking, we are still chasing our tails.

Over the years various syndromes have taken the blame for backpain. The most enduring has been the so-called 'slipped' disc but others have taken their share: arthritis, joint sprain, muscle spasm, muscle tear, pinched nerve, blood clot, twisted sacrum. The list is endless and invariably it is none of the above.

Against all odds, I find myself roused to hypothesise a new model for the breakdown of spines, simply because the present one is so lacking. To date, little has been ventured in mapping a sequence of decay from commonplace simple backaches, to the complex incurable ones. The conventional view has always seen spinal problems popping up at random—with no relationship to a pre-existing more benign disorder, and no part to play in creating a more serious one down the track. Getting a handle on the 'treatment' has been just as ramshackle and consequently a riotous variety of back therapies abound—from drastic surgery at one end to realigning the pull of muscles or off-loading suppressed birth traumas at the other.

In parts of this book I have made intuitive leaps of faith in explaining how the spine works, and how things deteriorate when a simple fault goes unchecked. You just have to bear with me; I am trying to establish links between known spinal mechanics and the broken down wrecks I see before me every day. In doing this, I posit myself halfway between what they say in the laboratory and what I see over and over again on the shop floor. I also speak with some trepidation, having been singed already by the wrath caused by daring to differ from established views.

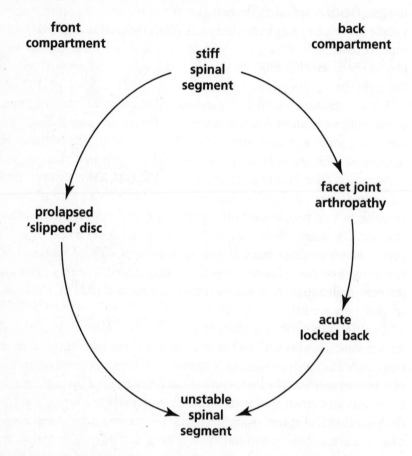

Diagram 1 The sequence of spinal breakdown.

THE WAY IT GOES WRONG...

I propose that a simple back pain develops when an intervertebral disc (the fibrous pillow between the vertebrae) loses water content and stiffens. This can be caused by several factors, not least small scale injury—either across or through the length of the spine—once the spine has become compressed. Then one of two things can happen for the problem to get worse: you can develop more serious trouble from the front compartment of the spine as the disc breaks down further. Or you can develop trouble from the back compartment as strain translates across to the facet joints. Worse still, you can get pain from both compartments at the same time. Finally, the wholesale destruction of both compartments can cause the vertebrae to jump around, in what is called segmental instability.

The sequential disorders in the route of breakdown is as follows:

Stage 1: A stiff spinal segment

An intervertebral disc between two vertebrae ceases to be a buoyant pillow and becomes like a layer of compressed carpet. The vertebra on top loses mobility and the segment becomes like a stiff link in the spinal chain. As it retires from activity the disc shrinks because it cannot generate sufficient suction to feed itself. Eventually the flattening can be picked up on X-ray, but well before this point the condition can be painful—in what I believe is the most common spinal disorder.

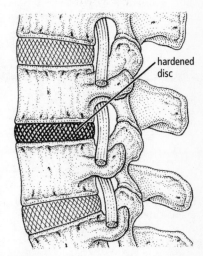

hardened disc

Figure 1 A stiff spinal segment is like a stiff link in a bicycle chain.

Stage 2: Arthritis of the facet joints

As a disc at the front of the spine drops in height it causes overriding of the bone-to-bone junctions (called the facet joints) at the back of the spine. The upper vertebra settles down on the one below, causing bony rub between parts of the spine which should only have fleeting contact. Early on, this simply inflames the soft tissues around the facet joints but eventually it causes arthritic change as it erodes the cartilage covering the bone. Facet joint trouble also is a relatively common form of low back pain.

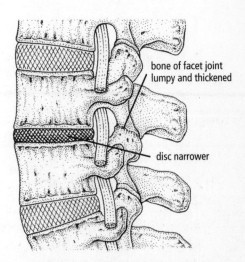

bone of facet joint lumpy and thickened

disc narrower

Figure 2 The wear and tear of facet joint arthropathy.

Stage 3: An acute locked back

This is a fluke incident when you are caught halfway through a movement by a pain like an electric cleaver going through your back. It makes moving in any direction excruciating and the body locks itself rigid. Although there never appears to be any warning, the problem usually has its origins in incipient disc breakdown.

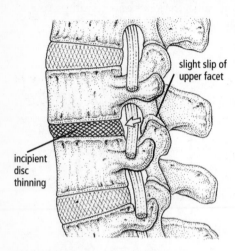

slight slip of upper facet

incipient disc thinning

Figure 3 A facet joint slipping askew in an acute locked back.

All spines, even healthy ones, must brace themselves as they pass through a vulnerable part of range at the beginning of a bending movement. If a disc between two vertebrae has flattened through the degenerative process, it may be unable to generate sufficient springing-apart tension to keep its segments stable as the spine goes over. The top vertebra can jump imperceptibly out of joint at one of the facets, and the muscles develop instantaneous protective spasm to stop the verterbra going any further.

Stage 4: A slipped disc

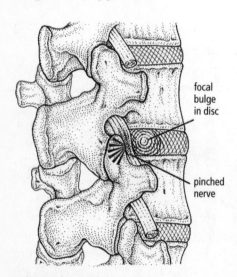

focal bulge in disc

pinched nerve

Figure 4 The focal bulge of a 'slipped' disc.

As a disc progressively loses its stuffing, it bulges like a perishing car tyre whenever it takes weight. The fibrous disc wall takes most of the strain, and in some cases it can perish at the points of greatest duress—usually one of the back corners. At the same time, the centre of the disc (called the nucleus) loses cohesion, after which excessive twisting and lifting activity can make it extrude through a fissure in the wall where it is weak. Sometimes the displaced nucleus lodges on a nearby spinal nerve and causes pain.

Stage 5: An unstable segment

With progressive loss of internal pressure, the disc cannot spring-load its vertebra when the spine bends. With each movement, it goes to shear forward at the problem link, tugging at its own walls as it goes. As it perishes, more strain is taken by the other main structure holding the segment together, the capsular ligaments of the facet joints at the same level. Eventually these ligaments stretch too, leaving the vertebra unstable to wobble about in the column.

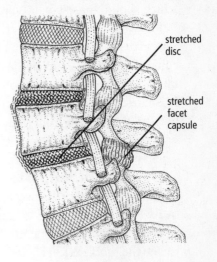

stretched disc

stretched facet capsule

In the event of severe arthritic change of the facets, instability can spread from the other side of the segment first. Eventually the disc suffers because stretched facet capsules allow too much movement of the segment. Frank instability of a segment is not a common cause of backpain—perhaps just as well, because it is exceedingly awkward to fix.

Figure 5 An unstable spinal segment is like a loose link in the chain.

THE WAY AHEAD...

The good news is that the right therapy almost anywhere along the route of spinal breakdown can stop it in its tracks and turn it around. Often curing a problem employs in reverse the same principles of destruction which brought it about in the first place. The linear progression through increasingly complex syndromes is just as straightforward in reverse.

The other good news is that you can do most of the rehabilitation yourself. Phase by less-painful phase you can steer yourself back out of the maze where you have been stumbling about for so long. At first you will barely believe it, or think you must be imagining things. Then in countless small ways you will feel your load lightening and your movements quickening. As you pass the hall table, you will pick up the newspaper on the run instead of planning every move. At last you will savour the sweet thrill of hope.

True, the passage of recovery may be far from smooth, and this is spelled out very clearly in the self-help sections of the book. The chapters on the various disorders contain suggested treatment regimens for the different phases, as well as actual case histories. The benefit of having both a hypothetical progression and an actual one is you see there is often a difference. You will also see there are occasional hiccups, even under the control of a therapist, which should make you less anxious if this happens to you.

Knowing how the spine works is critical, and for this reason there is quite a lot of detail in the book about spinal function. Seeing how it goes wrong is equally important, and by describing the symptoms of each disorder (as much as I specifically can) you are helped to know what your problem is. I also describe what I feel when I delve around in a back, and though this is not strictly relevant from your point of view, it throws more light on the wider picture. Remember, everything is much easier when you understand. Understanding is half the cure.

This book is designed to rescue sufferers from a wilderness of conflicting opinions and advice. However, there is no substitute for early hands-on treatment from a qualified therapist, preceded by careful diagnostic screening from a medical practitioner to exclude anything sinister. Your therapist will isolate the problem level, after which he or she will manually mobilise your spine to get the ball rolling. Then you will follow on with mobilising yourself, as well as stretching some muscle groups and strengthening others.

Knowing when to advance and when to backpedal on treatment is a grey area which is discussed. Even therapists find this difficult to gauge, and except for a specific knack using the hands, it is probably the one area which differentiates levels of skill. On the other hand, you on the 'inside' have instincts when treating yourself, which are a powerful ally. Keeping calm and in touch with your gut feelings, without being excessively introspective, will always steer you through a rough patch.

Ultimately, self treatment puts you in charge by making you responsible for your own back. It wrests you free of the endless rounds of appointments—going from one practitioner to the next—and takes you out of the passive patient role. It keeps you improving without being dependent, which means you are no longer the victim. Better still, it makes you the architect of your own destiny. It means…it's up to you!

1 How a normal spine works

This chapter describes the nuts and bolts of how the spine works. Parts of it are quite technical, particularly the mechanics of bending and the function of the various muscles, but I'm afraid there is no way of avoiding this. It is simply not possible to understand how things go wrong without first seeing how they should work. More to the point, the information lets you know what you are doing when it comes to fixing your back.

WHAT IS A SPINE?

The human spine is an upright bendy column. It consists of 24 separate segments called vertebrae which sit on top of each other in a vertical stack. There are seven in the neck (cervical), twelve in the middle back (thoracic) and five in the low back (lumbar). The base of the spine sits on the sacrum, which is a solid triangular block of bone at the back of the pelvis. The sacrum tilts down at the front to an angle of approximately 50 degrees below the horizontal, making a concavity in the low back as the spine arches to compensate.

The spine rises out of the pelvis in three gentle curves like a cobra from a basket. Its 'S' shape helps hold it upright, and by arching back and forth over a central line of gravity it balances the top-heavy torso over its narrow base. With perfect spinal alignment or posture, a straight line can be drawn through the ear, the tip of the shoulder, the spine at waist level, the knee joint and the back of the ankle.

The hollow in the low back is called a lumbar lordosis. This is followed by a gentle hump the other way in the chest region, called the thoracic kyphosis, and another arch in the neck called the cervical lordosis. The lumbar lordosis lessens with sitting when the pelvis tips backwards on the sitting bones (the ischial tuberosities) and increases with standing.

Perfect lumbar alignment achieves two important ends: it ensures the

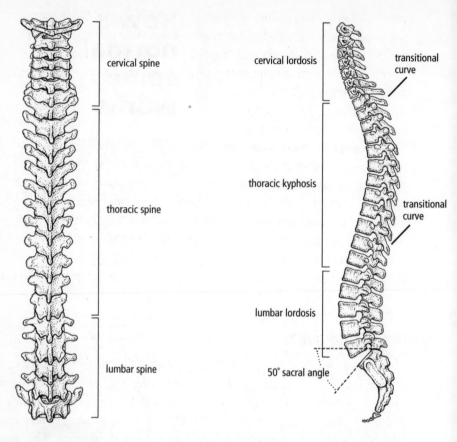

Figure 1.1 The human spine is a slender, segmented column made up of 24 vertebrae.

Figure 1.2 The forward slope of the sacrum determines the humping and hollowing of the spinal curves. Just the right amount of lumbar lordosis is a critical issue with backs.

correct distribution of body weight through the front and back compartment of the spine, and allows your low back to bow forward slightly to absorb impact during walking. As you might imagine, the right amount of lumbar lordosis is an important factor with backpain.

The following discussion highlights the anatomy which allows the spine to move in its free-flowing way—guiding it and controlling it so it doesn't go too far.

The lumbar vertebrae

The vertebrae are the individual building blocks of the spine. Each has a front and back compartment. The front compartment consists of the circular vertebral body, shaped like a cotton reel, which is specifically designed to stack easily and bear weight. The back compartment protects the spinal cord and hooks the spinal segments together so they stay in place.

Five lumbar vertebrae make up the low back. At the base of the spine the bottom vertebra (L5) sits on the sacrum and the junction between the two is called the lumbo-sacral or L5–S1 joint. As the most compressed level in the spine it is the most problematic. Nearly all low backpain comes from dysfunction of the front or back compartment (sometimes both) at this level.

The back compartment is a ring of bone extending backwards from the vertebral body which barely takes weight. In standing it bears approximately 16 per cent of bodyweight, but less if the spine is more humped in the sitting position where the facets are less engaged. With severe disc narrowing—the primary form of breakdown of the spine—the facets may be forced to take much more weight (up to 70 per cent of the weight through the spine), which is tremendously destructive.

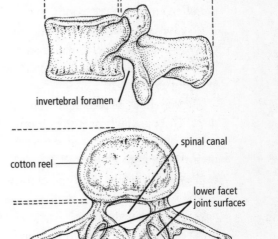

Figure 1.3 The vertical bodies of the front compartment are designed to stack easily and to bear weight, while the bony ring of the back compartment protects the cord and notches the spine together.

Each ring of the back compartment has small projections of bone sprigging from the outside corners: two wings out either side, called the transverse processes and a fin projecting out the back called the spinous process (these are the knobs of the spine running down the back you can see through the skin). All these bony bars serve as levers for the attachment of muscles which make the vertebrae move.

All the muscles working the segments exert a downward pull as they make them move. This is noteworthy because lumbar compression is the main cause of low backpain. If you bear in mind how much time we spend upright, fighting the weighing-down effects of gravity, you can see there are two factors at the start—our weight and the muscular strings moving the vertebrae—contributing to compression of the spine. There is also a third factor: the compression caused by sitting.

The cotton reels superimposed on one another at the disc–vertebra union make up the beautifully bendable neurocentral core, and the junctions between are often called the interbody joints. The bony inter-notching either side at the back makes a chain of mobile juicy aphophyseal or facet joints, running down the entire length of the spine. Together, the two different types of joints of the front and back compartment make up the total 'motion segment' at each spinal level.

The vertebrae are prevented from grinding on one other by the intervertebral discs. These are high-pressure fibrous sacks containing a central unsquashable sphere of mucoid fluid called a nucleus. The long column of bones with its high-tensile fibro-elastic pillows makes the neurocentral core thrusting and resilient, able to take nearly all of the weight passing down through the body.

The actual shape of the bodies of the vertebrae helps spread the load. They have a narrow waist which flares out to a broad weight-bearing upper and lower surface. Unlike the other lumbar vertebrae, L5 is thinner at the back which helps to form the lumbar lordosis. Its disc is also slightly wedge-shaped although it is still the fattest disc in the spine, helping it to bear the load of the rest of the spine on top.

Each 'cotton reel' is made up of a layer of hard cortical bone on the outside and honeycomb bone (called cancellous bone) on the inside. This is sometimes called the 'spongiosa' because it resembles a sponge and stores a rich supply of blood. The presence of the blood inside the bones is ingenious when it comes to dispersing forces through the bone.

Apart from being a handy reservoir, the fluid inside helps absorb the impact of shock passing through the vertebrae. These box-like bodies, literally bursting with blood, transmit the forces of compression in all directions throughout the fluid,

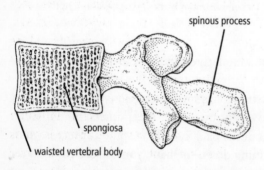

spinous process

spongiosa

waisted vertebral body

Figure 1.4 The honeycomb bone of the spongiosa is really a three-dimensional scaffold which stops the bone crumbling under pressure. The blood reservoirs in the vertebrae help absorb shock.

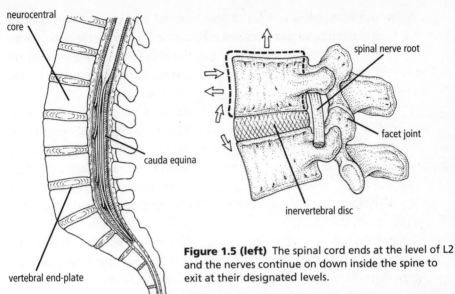

neurocentral core

cauda equina

vertebral end-plate

spinal nerve root

facet joint

inervertebral disc

Figure 1.5 (left) The spinal cord ends at the level of L2 and the nerves continue on down inside the spine to exit at their designated levels.

Figure 1.6 (above) The vertebral bodies roll around on their disc while the facets at the back act like 'guide rails' to keep the movement in check.

thereby dissipating the direct downward pressure. As well as reducing strain, this functions as a useful engine for shunting nutrients into the disc, which does not have its own blood supply.

The line of demarcation between the vertebra and the upper and lower surfaces of the disc is called the vertebral end-plate. It is a thin cartilaginous interface about 1 mm thick and although each one is cushioned by the disc in between, it is still the weakest part of the spine. With rigorous impact, each end-plate can seem like a semi-destructible membrane caught between two thundering fluid-transmitted systems: the vertebral body on one side and the disc on the other. Sometimes, impact through the spine can blow a tiny vent in an end-plate, like blowing a hole through hide stretched over a drum.

The honeycomb bone inside the vertebra is actually a gridwork of tiny struts and spars, like an internal scaffolding. Its three-dimensional structure prevents the roof of the vertebra caving in and the walls collapsing inwards like a cardboard box being flattened. It is a brilliant way of making the bones strong yet light. If the vertebrae were solid it would be much harder for our spines to operate. Not only would the bone tend to cleave off in chunks when subjected to compression and torsional strains but we would hardly be able to move for our own weight.

When the vertebrae are superimposed on one another, the consecutive bony rings at the back make a hollow tube inside the spine called the spinal canal. The canal houses the fragile spinal cord of the central nervous system which hangs down from the base of the brain like a long plait of hair. Filaments of nervous tissue branch off either side all the way down and become the spinal nerve roots. The cord itself actually ends at the level of the second lumbar vertebra. The roots then continue on inside the spine, hanging down like strands of a horse's tail (hence the name *cauda equina*) until they make their exit either side through their designated inter-segmental level.

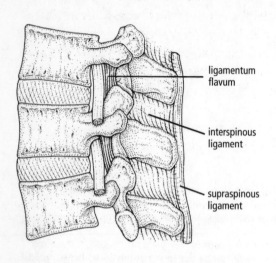

ligamentum flavum

interspinous ligament

supraspinous ligament

Figure 1.7 The 'posterior ligamentous lock' generates greatest tension when the back is round; this makes it easy to see why we should lift with a bent back.

Whereas the role of the front compartment is fairly straightforward as a weight-bearing strut, the workings of the back compartment are more complex. Apart from acting as casing to protect the spinal cord it has two other important functions: to guide the movement of the vertebrae—favouring some and keeping other more troublesome ones to a minimum—and helping to lock the vertebrae together to stop them slipping off one another.

The spinal ligaments

The spinal ligaments are a very important backup system in keeping the spinal segments together. Between the bony locking mechanism and the muscular system they guide and restrain the movements of the vertebrae. The most important group is 'the posterior ligamentous system' made up of the ligamentum flavum, the interspinous and the supraspinous ligaments. They make a festoonery of reinforced fibrous bands joining up the bony levers at the back of the spine and reinforcing the capsular ligaments. The whole system comes into its own when the spine has to lift.

The ligamentum flavum is a thick short ligament covering the front of the facet joints at each segmental level. Each one has a smooth surface to help create a flawless, comfortable lining for the back of the spinal canal with its delicate neural matter inside.

In its healthy state the ligamentum flavum is an unusual ligament because it has more muscle tissue (elastin 80 per cent) than fibrous (collagen 20 per cent), making it in reality a 'muscular' ligament. While the ligamentum flavum covers the front of the facet joints, the multifidus muscle (about which you will read a great deal in this book) covers the back. With both muscles right at the nexus of forward movement of a segment, they are intimately involved in controlling it. In particular they guard the laxity of the facet joints—which are the most likely part of the spine to come undone. They stand like sentries front and back, controlling how much they pay out to let facets open so the spine can bend.

Both 'muscles' do an equally important job during bending: through the facets they generate a tension on the back of the interspace, which pressurises the disc. This primes or pre-tenses it, which stops any unwanted wobble of the segment as the spine goes over. It is a vitally important role and you will see in Chapter 4 how sometimes it slips up. If the spine goes to bend before it has worked up sufficient holding power in multifidus—usually by bending with a weak tummy and the back arched instead of humped—there can be a fluke mishap where the vertebra jumps out of joint.

The interspinous ligament and the supraspinous ligament have a less pivotal role to play. They come into their own as a steadfast ligamentous lock down the back of your spine when the low back is fully humped. As such, they play an intimate part of a proper lifting technique which (contrary to what you may have heard) can only work if the back starts off round. The interspinous ligament is situated between the tails of the vertebrae with its fibres aligned in such a way that they resist the pulling open of the vertebrae. The supraspinous ligament runs from tip to tip of the spinous processes (the tails) and also helps them to resist splaying open. There is no supraspinous ligament between L5–S1 interspace, presumably because this is taken care of by the massively strong ilio-lumbar ligament.

The ilio-lumbar ligament provides the main shoring for the base of the spine. It is a broad star-shaped band of fibrous thickening which passes from the inside bowl either side of the pelvis and converges upwards on the lowest vertebra, attaching itself strongly through the two huge transverse processes which curve downwards to meet it like tusks.

Incidentally, to provide extra strength in lashing the base of the spine to the sacral table, the transverse processes of L5 are built in a pyramidal shape with a broader base to receive the two strong ropes of the ilio-lumbar ligament.

Handy as this may be in providing a better base for attachment, it does somewhat occlude the diameter of the intervertebral foraminae. These are the two small holes below the transverse processes at every spinal level through which the nerve roots issue. If you bear in mind that the L5 root is also the thickest, you can start to see why it is so prone to being inflamed by pathological processes affecting either the front or back compartment (or both) of the lumbar-sacral level.

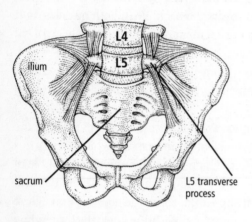

Figure 1.8 The wide-spreading ilio-lumbar ligament lashes the base of the spine to the sacrum.

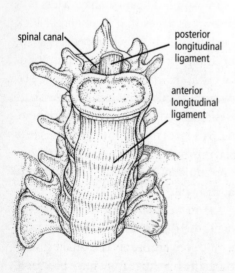

Figure 1.9 The strap-like anterior and posterior longitudinal ligaments bind the front and back of the cotton reels in a ligamentous strait-jacket.

The long tube of cotton reels making up the neurocentral core is reinforced front and back by two strap-like ligaments called the anterior and posterior longitudinal ligaments. The anterior longitudinal ligament is the strongest ligament in the spine and by interlinking with the front of the vertebrae it stops your spine bending back too far. It also prevents the lower back sinking too deeply into an arch (or lordosis) as the spine takes weight.

The posterior longitudinal ligament runs down the back of the cotton reels, spreading out over the back of each disc in a cross-hatched arrangement of fibres to reinforce the back wall. Significantly, it can be irritated by a disc squeezing out between its two vertebrae in the case of a prolapsed intervertebral disc (see Chapter 5). More than the other ligaments, it has a highly developed nerve supply and is extremely sensitive to being stretched by bulging disc material.

The intervertebral disc

At its simplest, the spine gets most of its movement from each cotton reel sitting on its discal pillow and careening about in all directions. The back compartment has to control that movement.

The intervertebral discs are the pillows and they are vital to the spine. Their high bursting pressure thrusts the vertebrae apart while at the same time gluing them together. Each has a vigorous incompressibility, like standing on a breadboard balanced on a beachball. They give the spine a quivering up-thrusting romp which makes it whippy and light so it can tip around freely in the air without flopping over like a broken reed.

Each disc consists of a squirting liquid centre called the nucleus and a tough meshed outer wall called the annulus fibrosis. The annulus in turn is made up of approximately twelve thin fibrous layers (called lamellae) which make up the wall. For maximum strength in bending each successive lamellae is made of fibres running in diagonally opposing directions, like the walls of a radial car tyre. This creates a tenacious multi-layered tubular lattice running around the rim of the disc which is bonded strongly to the vertebrae above and below. Thus the disc wall not only holds the vertebrae firmly together; it also keeps the nucleus under pressure.

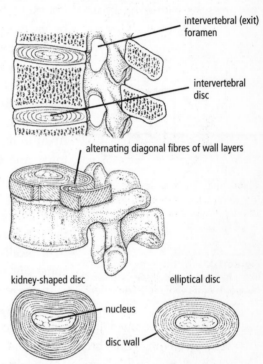

Figure 1.10 Each disc consists of a liquid pearl nucleus and a tough multi-layered wall which keeps the nucleus under pressure and bonds the vertebrae together.

The lamellae at the back of the disc are even thinner and bunched closely together. This gives the interspaces more freedom to pull apart so the spine can bend forward—its most frequent act—but it also means it is weaker, introducing a precarious trade-off between freedom to bend and the possibility that over-bending could break down the wall.

Often the L5 discs are kidney-shaped, which exposes a longer flank and increases the holding power of the back wall. However, kidney-shaped discs have the disadvantage of runkling more in the acute back corners when torsion strains are applied to the disc. You will see later how heavy duty lifting and twisting actions can make the wall perish at these points.

The nucleus of the disc has a unique molecular make-up which allows it to attract fluid to keep itself hydrated under pressure. (When healthy nuclear material is taken from a disc and set in a saucer of fluid it swells by 300 per cent.) This powerful attractive force from the nucleus maintains the high pressures within the disc so it is not squashed dry, as a normal sponge would be, by the powerful and ever-present forces bearing down upon it.

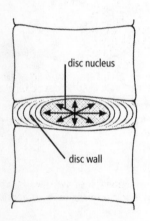

disc nucleus

disc wall

Figure 1.11 The disc's nucleus acts like a hydraulic sack, dispersing forces outwards and evenly in all directions.

When a disc is young, the nucleus is nearly 90 per cent water but as it gets older it is less able to hold it. Even so, the strong suction on water creates very high intradiscal pressures. Apart from making the disc unsquashable, it forces the disc walls outwards, which has ingenious benefits for the spine. The strength of the walls fighting back against the outward force stiffens them and gives each link between the vertebrae invaluable tensile strength. This dynamically braces each link and keeps the spine taut all the way down its length.

In the world of physics, a disc operating like this is called an 'hydraulic sack'. Compression of a contained fluid results in forces being distributed outwards and evenly in all directions through that fluid. In the realm of backs, this is very important and the fluid content of any disc is critical to its high performance.

Our vertical posture enhances the tensile strength of the spine. It adds to the pressurising of the fluid sacks and converts the spine into a spring-loaded rod which can flip up straight again after bending. Without these tensile properties, the human back would not be the long slender thing it is. We would need a hugely bulky muscular apparatus to haul us up straight again once we had doubled over.

But vertical posture does have its down side. It means the segments at the bottom of the stack get squashed by carrying so much weight. Compression down through the spine is the single most important cause of low back pain.

The vertebral movements

The movements of the vertebrae in the spine are a combination of gliding, tipping and twisting, although each one individually contributes only a small degree. Superimposed one on one however, the net result is the grandiose wide-ranging mobility of the spine, which is so well-known to us. From our towering height we can arch backwards under a limbo bar and bend over to cut our toenails. Well, some of us can.

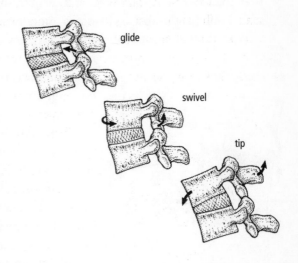

Of the vertebral movements, gliding is the least generous. The upper vertebra slides transversely forwards, backwards and from side to side on the vertebra below but the actual distances travelled are minute. Glide is more of a background move-

Figure 1.12 All the vertebrae glide, swivel and tip to a small degree, but together, overall spinal movement is grandiose.

ment which better positions the vertebra for action; it sets the stage and puts the vertebra at its optimum starting point for the more adventurous tipping and twisting activity to follow.

As we bend to touch our toes, for example, each vertebra moves forward incrementally on the one below, bringing the upper one to its perfect starting point for tipping. The element of glide contributes the typical flowing quality to the way all living creatures move (a cheetah on the run has it in spades). Without it, all living actions are much more clipped and jerky and not nearly as streamlined and expansive. An elderly lady tottering along the footpath has very little glide in her joints.

The right amount of vertebral glide is important; it is what healthy backs have. Too little or too much glide leads to trouble. If a segment has too little it will be stiff. Significantly, when the degenerative process sets in, this is the first movement to go. Although you cannot necessarily see it—first you only feel it—this lack of background movement makes your spine feel tighter; more restricted and laboured in everything it does. In short it makes you feel rigid and 'older' than you are.

At the other extreme, a vertebral segment is unstable if it has too much glide. It comes to light when the spine bends over and the top vertebra slips forward on the lower one. This is known as segmental instability, and it actually stems from stiffness of a segment. What distinguishes the former from the latter is the total degeneration of the motion segment. It is the stuff of this book and is discussed step by step throughout.

With normal segmental mobility, all the vertebrae roll around on their liquid ball bearing discs whose fibrous walls keep everything in place. As the upper vertebra moves off-centre, tension takes up in the wall mesh and brakes the action. And as soon as bend is incorporated into the action, another brake comes on from the squirting pressure of the nucleus.

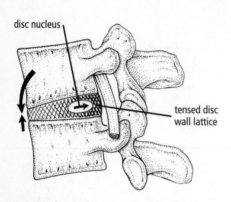

Figure 1.13 The bending action invokes its own brake when the backward migration of the nucleus makes the back wall of the disc taut; this makes it harder for the vertebrae to pull apart.

With bending forward, which is our most repeated action, the nucleus is squidged towards the back of the disc. Were it not for the toughness of the wall, the distortion would make it balloon out backwards. But because the wall is so strong, most of the force is taken up or absorbed by it. Thus the intradiscal pressure adds extra stiffening to the mesh. In this pre-stiffened state it then retards the gapping of the two adjacent vertebrae as they try to pull apart with bending. The tensioned mesh slows the rate at which the back of the vertebrae can separate and steadies the bending.

The nutrition of the disc

The intervertebral disc has no blood supply so it keeps alive by other means. It relies heavily on push-me pull-me forces through the spine to shunt fluids in and out of the discs through the end-plates from the rich capillary beds in the neighbouring vertebral bodies. Apart from the molecular suction generated by the nuclear gel with its strong pull on water, routine pressure changes on the spine greatly enhance the tidal flow of fluids in and out of the disc.

As the spine pulls out, like an elongated concertina, nutrients and oxygen are sucked into the discs. As the spine squashes down again, carbon dioxide and metabolites are pushed back out through the end-plates. Thus a dynamic pump is provided by routine spinal activity, no matter how humble the task.

As you bend down to the washing basket the lumbar discs are loaded, which forces fluids out. As you reach up to hang the clothes over the line the reduced pressure sucks fresh fluids back in.

The more grandiose and varied the movement, the more efficient the imbibition pump is. The more active the spine, the more marked the alterations of the pressure inside the discs. This improves the fluid exchange and keeps the discs puffed up. Flamboyant movement (with as little jarring impact as possible) keeps the spine young; it gives the discs a drink. It creates a natural ebb and flow of nutrients in and out which is vital for their ongoing health.

Sadly, one of the oldest directives in the management of bad backs

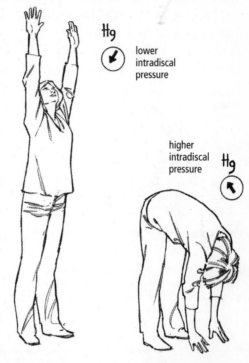

Figure 1.14 Bending over raises the intradiscal pressure which shunts fluid out, while stretching up lessens the pressure which sucks fluid in. Thus the disc acquires a 'circulation'.

hampers disc nutrition. Even today people the world over are being told never to bend, especially if their back hurts. Since the days when slipped discs hijacked the debate on backs, everybody has heard (including me as a young physiotherapist) that bending could make a disc pop out, which might pinch a nerve. You will see that things just don't work this way. The notion in the first place is the product of misguided imagination.

I place enormous importance in this book on bending, and the understanding of its mechanics. Eventually you will agree it is not only quite useful to bend, but vital for the ongoing health of your spine—and for the treatment of a weak and stiff back once it has become painful. You will see how learning to bend makes a bad back healthy again. You will also see that far from causing damage, bending is essentially normal and very important.

The facet joints

These are the junctions formed where the vertebrae notch together at the back of the spine. Each motion segment has two facet joints forming part of the back compartment. They flank the back corners of each disc, across the gulf of the vertebral canal.

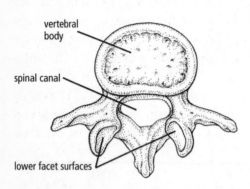

Figure 1.15 Two facet joints flank the back corners of each disc across the gulf of the spinal canal.

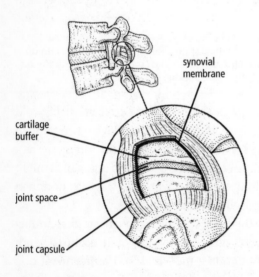

Figure 1.16 The opposing cartilage-covered surfaces of each facet fit together like two palms pressed together.

Neighbouring vertebrae contribute two opposing surfaces to make a pair of facet joints. Two notches of bone project up from the lower vertebral ring interfacing with two projecting down from the upper vertebral ring. Thus two inter-notching junctions are made.

The facet joints do not bear a lot of weight unless the disc is thin or the lumbar lordosis extreme, but they suffer constant wear and tear in controlling the movement of their vertebra. To protect the joint surfaces a properly functioning joint needs to exist where the two bones meet.

The most capable and resilient joints in the body are synovial joints, and all of them—whether in the fingers, knees or facet joints—share common properties. They have extremely strong joint capsules which knit the two sides of the joint together. The capsules have a well-wired nervous network to make the joint highly sensitive and they also have a prolific blood supply. The inner lining of the capsules (called the synovial membrane) floods the joint with synovial fluid which both dampens impact and lubricates the working surfaces.

The facet joint capsules are

unusually strong. With bending forward they provide nearly as much soft-tissue restraint as the discs in gluing the spinal segments together. Researchers have removed the discs from cadavers in a laboratory and shown that almost twice bodyweight can be suspended by the facet capsules alone. Thus they are more than simple joint capsules: they are more like ligaments and for this reason they take the name 'capsular ligaments'.

Each facet joint has a smooth-interfacing congruency of its opposing joint surfaces. These fit snugly together like two cupped palms, the valleys of one side matching the hills on the other. The surfaces of the opposing bones are covered by hyaline cartilage which is a smooth semi-compliant buffer with a rich mother-of-pearl sheen.

Cartilage allows the bones to skid over one another and has the yielding consistency of dense plastic which allows it to deform imperceptibly whenever the bones make contact. The direct contact also squeezes fluid out, but when the pressure releases and the cartilage un-dints, it sucks water back in. In this way the bloodless cartilage keeps itself healthy by creating a 'circulation' to pull in nutrients and expel waste products.

The slippery cartilage interfaces are lubricated by synovial fluid just as tears flush the eyes and this synovial fluid has astonishing qualities of lightness and slipperiness. The joint capsule keeps the fluid contained under pressure that springs the joint surfaces apart and softens the impact of bone on bone. It also means the joint operates on a cushion of fluid (in an hydraulic sack) which streamlines movement and takes out the jerkiness.

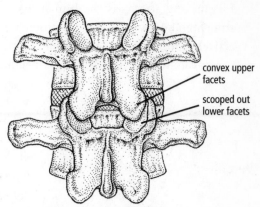

convex upper facets

scooped out lower facets

Synovial fluid also cleanses the joint space by clearing away cartilage particles eroded off the main bed during activity. The synovial membrane liberates large cartilage-eating cells into the tide of floating debris. These cells surround each particle, like an amoeba trapping its food, and dissolve it. It is es-

Figure 1.17 The cupped bowl of the lower facet surfaces notches the vertebrae together and facilitates forward bending only.

sential cleaning-up work. Without it the joints would silt up with cartilaginous grit acting like a pot-scourer, grinding away the joint surfaces until nothing was left.

The chain of facet joints down the spine provide a primitive interlinking hook-up which notches the spinal segments together. The upper facet surfaces are convex and the lower ones concave. This allows the upper vertebrae to lock in place when its convex pillars fit snugly into the concave cups of the ones below.

If the facets were not there the vertebrae could roll around on their discs and the neurocentral core could tie itself in knots like a cartoon character of an India-rubber man. However, the definite front-back alignment of the lumbar facets means our only generous movement of the low back is bending forward. Their configuration means the vertebrae only move forward and back, like the wheels of a train moving down the track, never twisting left or right (although they can side-bend a little). This lets us lower the rest of our body down, like a stooping mechanical crane, putting our hands and face at the right height to be useful.

There is good reason for the facets otherwise restricting movement: it keeps things from wearing out. The twisting action in the low back is especially hard on the discs. It challenges the inherent weakness of their walls, especially if there is lifting as well. With only every alternate layer of the onion-skin disc wall offering restraint (while the fibres of the other half go on the slack offering no help), repeated twisting can be destructive.

The bending human spine

Elegant and strong as the human back is, the job of bending over and straightening up again is a tall order. The trunk and spinal muscles which actively control the movement are discussed further on. However, several other anatomical features help make bending possible, by working as a physical brake to control the free fall of the spine when it tips forward.

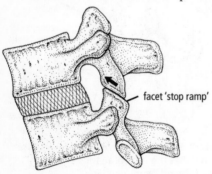

facet 'stop ramp'

The first of these we have discussed already: the strong fibrous wall of the disc which binds the cotton reels together. This contributes about 29 per cent to the control of the segments going forward. As the segments glide forward the stiff fibrous mesh of the wall retards the initial movement. When the spinal segments then tip forward and the back of the interspaces open up, the same diagonal mesh pulls up, like stretching up a garden lattice.

Figure 1.18 As the spine bends, the vertebrae slide up the 'stop-ramps' increasing the tension between the segments and making the back more secure.

However, even more important in controlling bend are the various structures of the back compartment. The facets contribute in two ways: a sloping stop-ramp, made by the joint surfaces, and extremely tough capsular ligaments. When viewed from the side, the lower facet surfaces taper upwards towards the front of the spine. As the spine bends this means the upper vertebrae must travel uphill as they go forward.

(They work like emergency stop-ramps beside steep downhill sections of highways, gradually bringing the vehicle to a halt as it nears the top of the ramp.)

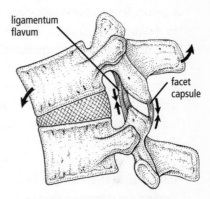

ligamentum flavum

facet capsule

In the case of the back, the escalating tension of the soft tissues gradually brings the upper vertebra to a halt, by which time the facet interfaces are firmly locked against each another and the ligamentum flavum and the facet capsule are tense at full stretch. It is a marvellously ingenious system with both bone and soft tissue complementing the workings of each other.

Figure 1.19 When we round our backs to bend, maximum tension is generated in both the ligamentum flavum and the facet capsules, thus holding the segments stable.

As we go further into a bend the upper vertebra then tips bodily forward by pivoting on the front edge, as the tail of the vertebra attempts to lift away. This second part of the movement is restrained mainly by the facet joint capsules. They contribute a powerful 39 per cent towards moderating bending. The ligamentum flavum contributes an initial 13 per cent. All up, the facets contribute 52 per cent of

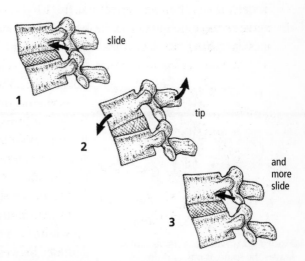

slide

tip

and more slide

1

2

3

Figure 1.20 With so few mechanisms to prevent shear, it is safest to bend forward with a round back to invoke all the mechanisms which control tip. By controlling tip, we control shear.

the ligamentous restraint on forward bending. No wonder they can suspend twice the body's weight.

It is very significant that none of these facet ligaments exert control over the forward *gliding* action of the segments, only forward tipping. Control of forward gliding is important because it is this action carried out to excess (when it is called forward shear) which constitutes the unstable element of a segment's movement. All segments must avoid shear, because it is potentially so devastating. And it is failure to control the forward tipping which allows too much shear. The process works like this:

As bending starts the initial forward glide is only about 2 mm before the facets engage to stop it. As the bend continues, the facets disengage with the tipping forward action which makes the tail of the vertebra lift up and away, leaving a gap between the two facet surfaces. However, once the tail of the vertebra is away, the whole vertebra can glide forward more, until the bony block engages once again. In this way, more tip allows more glide. Incidentally, the tipping action is what both the facet capsules and the ligamentum flavum are designed to resist, while multifidus, the deepest intrinsic muscle of the spine, is designed to control it actively.

The spinal nerves

In the lumbar area, the nerve roots emerge from the spine under their corresponding vertebra. Thus the left and right L1 nerve roots come out under the first lumbar vertebra at the L1–2 interspace and so on. The L5 nerve roots come out at the lumbo-sacral junction. The spinal nerves carry messages to the muscles to make the legs work and also carry sensory messages back inside, relaying information from the outside world back to the brain.

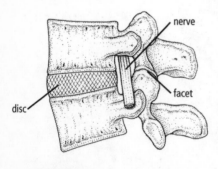

Figure 1.21 When the nerve root leaves the spine, it passes right between the disc sucking and billowing on one side and the facet capsules tugging and puckering on the other— a precarious arrangement!

As the nerve roots leave the spine they travel out through small canals (called the intervertebral foraminae) bordered on one side by the facet joint and on the other by the disc. It is less than ideal to have these fragile strands of nervous tissue making their exit right through the machinery of a complex human hinge. It means they run the gauntlet between the very two structures most likely to cause trouble in the spine.

As each nerve root goes about its business, it has the intervertebral disc sucking and billowing on one side and the facet joint with its baggy capsule tugging and puckering on the other. The nerve is largely protected from these goings on by a protective sleeve or nerve sheath which extends just beyond the spine, like the cuff of a shirt poking out from a coat.

As you will read in the next chapter, pathological change of either the disc or facet joint can cause thickening, hardening and swelling. By direct contact, the inflammation can spread to the nerve root, simply because it is so close. Inflammation of the nerve causes severe pain down the leg, known as sciatica.

The muscles which work the spine

As superbly designed as the spine is, it amounts to nought without the dynamic contribution of the muscles. In the way a puppet is a flummoxed pile of sticks on the floor without its strings, the human spine and its segments is an inert, toppling pole without its muscles.

The muscles of the human body work just like the strings of a puppet. They pull on levers and make the body move. They allow us to keep the thinking, acting, top part of the body up there so we can operate effectively in the outside world. Without the dynamic support of the muscles the spine would fall over. More than you would ever imagine, the muscles play a

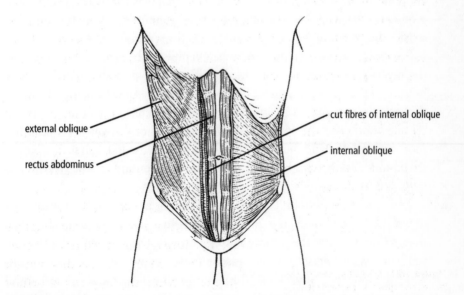

external oblique

rectus abdominus

cut fibres of internal oblique

internal oblique

Figure 1.22 The rectus abdominus muscle runs down the front of the abdomen, whereas the internal and external obliques cross over each other diagonally, creating the enviable 'wasp' waist.

dynamically synchronised role in keeping the skeleton upright and controllable.

You only have to see unfortunate cases of poliomyelitis to understand this point. With paralysis of the trunk muscles, the spine tumbles down around itself in slow motion, like a collapsing circular staircase, with the chest disappearing into the abdomen and into the pelvis. The tummy muscles play a critical role in keeping the towering spine up there.

Tummy muscles also play a critical role in letting the spine bend. Although there is some confusion about the mechanism by which this happens, practising therapists the world over recognise the importance of a strong tummy in treating back problems. Still today, researchers cannot agree about the best way to strengthen these muscles. I certainly have my ideas which you will read about later in the book.

The abdominal muscles spread vertically, horizontally and diagonally, wrapping the soft abdomen in sheets of contractile tissue. As they contract, their fibres shorten and bow the spine forward. Working statically they nip in the waist, creating the 'hourglass' figure and flattening the belly. This effect reduces the intra-abdominal space, which automatically raises the intra-abdominal pressure.

A strong tummy stabilises the spine from in front, in several ways. Firstly, a strong co-contraction with the back muscles lifts the spine vertically. This is similar to the upward movement of water in a plastic bottle if you grasp it around the waist. (If the bottle has no lid the contents spurt out the top.) The tension between the segments increases as the spine grows longer.

Secondly, a strong abdominal contraction pulls the belly in, slightly humping the low back and creating a contained pocket of high intra-abdominal pressure in front of the spine, like an air bag in a car. Apart from stiffening the spine, the back pressure against the lumbar segments prevents them shearing forward on one another as the spine bends. As the bend of the low back becomes more accentuated and the tails of the vertebrae fan out like fish scales flaring, the posterior ligaments achieve their maximum tension and create a ligamentous lock. At this point the spine becomes more stable.

As we bend, the abdominal muscles and their opposite number, the muscles down the back of the spine, help in a coordinated way to lower the spine over. From the front the tummy muscles provide the hydraulics for the fine precision. With fantastic, noiseless accuracy they allow us to adjust our height, while the long back muscles let the spine go, like the cables of a mechanical crane paying out. They particularly come into their own around the hoop of the spine when we are nearly at full bend. What a beautiful system the working spine is!

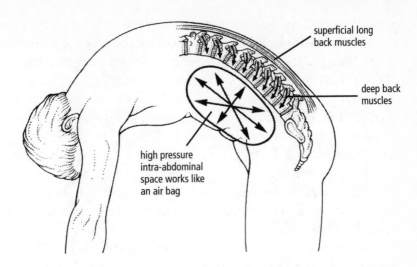

Figure 1.23 When straightening, both the long back muscles and the small intrinsics work best around the hoop of the spine—this explains why you must always come up with a tight tummy and a round back.

Whether the bend is great or small, lowering the top-heavy column and then straightening it is a stupendously difficult task, especially when accompanied by lifting. Some mathematical calculations suggest the smallness of the back muscles and the awkward angles make it impossible, particularly if lifting is also involved. Since we all know that our spines do bend and lift, and fairly effortlessly at that (though some better than others), we at least must concede the working spine is an awesomely effective thing.

With bending, the muscles of the spine and trunk work in two distinct ways: they centrally clench the segments together to keep them stable, and then they control the lowering over of the whole column. This vertical clenching of the spine is an important preparatory contribution to stability, while the bending itself is almost free fall. Rather than actually doing anything, the main job of the muscles is keeping control as the column goes over, so nothing comes undone.

Weakness in the central clamping down action is one of the earliest things to go wrong with a back once it starts to break down. We do not know yet why this is so; whether it is a case of cause or effect. In other words, we cannot say whether the muscles reflexly inhibit once there *is* inflammation between segments, or whether the inflammation develops because there is weakness of the muscles keeping the segments together.

Coming up from the bend the whole process works in reverse. While the spine is still stooped, the ligamentous lock holds it stable and the unfurling

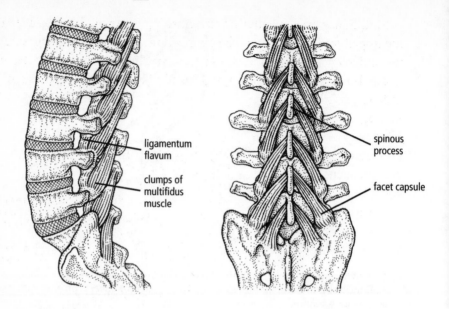

Figure 1.24 The deep layers of multifidus originate on the spinous process two vertebrae above and then pass down and laterally to insert on the back of the facet capsules.

starts by the pelvis rolling back. Then the static tensing of the abdomen thrusts us up from in front and the intrinsic muscles of the spine work at segmental level pulling each vertebra back. The large superficial muscles work around the hoop of the spine when we are in full bend, and then again like guy ropes once we are upright.

Multifidus is intimately in control of bend—especially in the early part of range—and is the most important intrinsic spinal muscle. It originates either side of the spine, on the bony ring of the back compartment, right over the top of the facet joints. It is the deepest segmental muscle and its fibres actually blend in with the back of the facet capsules (which is significant with facet trouble, see Chapters 3 and 4). The fibres then pass upwards and inwards to the vertebra two above where they attach themselves to the spinous process. With the spine upright the line of pull of multifidus fibres is at 90 degrees (or right angles) to the spinous process it is attached to. Thus it is optimally placed to control the segments at the very first glimmer of bending.

In straightening from the bent-over position, multifidus initially gets a bit of help from the 'muscular' ligament, the ligamentum flavum, each working its own side of the joint. The smaller front muscle tries to close the joint by sliding the two joint surfaces together, while the larger multifidus closes the gap by pulling on the tail at the back of the spine.

Multifidus's main role during straightening is to pull down on the tail of the tipped-forward vertebra, like pulling down an overhead garage door. As we straighten, the spine unfurls step by step in a segmental fashion, from the hooped-over position to fully upright. Multifidus is vitally important in controlling instability of the spinal segments, and it works hand in glove with the important stabiliser of the front compartment, transversus abdominus.

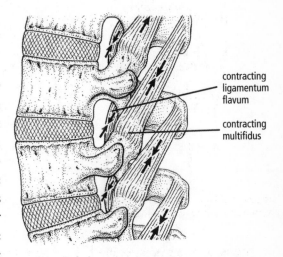

contracting ligamentum flavum

contracting multifidus

Multifidus does another unique job as it helps the spine straighten. It hoists the facet capsules out of the way, rather like a damsel gathering up her petticoats as she goes to climb the stairs. This prevents the tender capsular lining being nipped as the opposing surfaces close down when the spine straightens. As you will read in Chapter 4, sometimes the muscle's co-ordination is

Figure 1.25 When straightening, both ligamentum flavum and multifidus work right at the centre of movement, so are intimately involved in keeping the segment secure.

caught off guard and the capsule gets painfully jammed in the works. It is thought that the 'muscular' ligamentum flavum does a similar thing on the other side of the joint and prevents the baggy capsule getting nipped as the spine bends forward.

The other intrinsic muscles, iliocostalis and longissimus, control the forward shear of the vertebrae although they operate at a more difficult angle when the spine is more deeply bent forward. Their fibres pass in a direction closer to a back-front alignment. As the spine straightens they slide the vertebrae backwards in a reverse shearing action, rather like sliding drawers out of a chest.

The deepest tummy muscle, transversus abdominus, plays a unique role as it helps the spine straighten, because it works both as a tummy and back muscle at the same time. It originates from either side of the tummy, below the navel, passes transversely around the waist like a cummerbund and joins a sheet of fibrous tissue at the back called the thoraco-lumbar fascia. The fibres of the fascial sheet make a diagonal lattice which attaches in different layers to both the transverse and spinous processes of the lumbar vertebrae.

As the muscle contracts it creates a high pressure air bag in front of the spine (like any other tummy muscle). But it also tugs sideways on the thoraco-lumbar lattice. As the lattice pulls out laterally it becomes shallower in height which telescopes the cotton reels down on one another and tugs down on the tails of the vertebrae, thus clenching the spine.

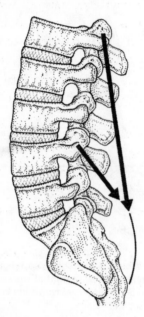

Figure 1.26 The direction of pull of iliocostalis and longissimus helps slide the vertebrae backwards as the spine straightens.

As well as helping multifidus regulate forward bending, transversus abdominus performs the very important role of clamping of the spinal segments together in preparation for spinal activity. This ensures the spine doesn't jump out of joint as soon as other movements pull it about. This clamping works in all sorts of ways, from the subtle to the spectacular. For instance, it gathers up the spinal segments and allows us to turn over in bed at night without waking, but it also stiffens your spine automatically as you see the tennis ball coming at you over the net. It converts the segments into a stiff lumbar pillar in anticipation for other things it has to do. With its tendency to get weak, no wonder these actions (to name but a few) are so painful with bad backs.

Recent research suggests that transversus abdominus is supported in keeping the segments stable by the ever-acting breathing muscle, the diaphragm. In an example of Nature's expediency, both take turn about in keeping the lateral tension on the thoraco-lumbar fascia. Since we breathe all the time I cannot imagine a better partner. What could be more appropriate than harnessing the breathing mechanism to assist another equally fundamental mechanism: keeping the central strut of the body intact.

It happens like this: The diaphragm attaches in part to the sides of the thoraco-lumbar fascia. It is a huge dome of contractile tissue which separates the thorax and abdomen, making both into watertight compartments. We take a breath in when the diaphragm contracts and flattens and descends in the chest. This increases the volume in the chest cavity but lowers the pressure, causing air to flow in through the nose. The contracting diaphragm tugs laterally on the sides of the thoraco-lumbar fascia, making each in-breath telescope the lumbar segments. As we breathe in, the low back is kept secure as we go about our business.

When it is time to breathe out the diaphragm relaxes, raising the pressure inside the chest compared to the outside, making air flow out. At the same time, the diaphragm hands over the reins to transversus abdominus which is active during the breathing out phase, but which also exerts tension on the thoraco-lumbar fascia. During expiration it shrinks the girth which automatically raises the intra-abdominal pressure, helping to stabilise the spine.

Thus with each 'muscle' taking turns to keep the thoraco-lumbar fascia tense, we keep our backs stable just by breathing. This also explains why it so often hurts to cough with a bad back. The explosive exhalation happens with a strong involuntary contraction of the tummy which jerks the thoraco-lumbar fascia sideways. This bounces the vertebrae vertically and

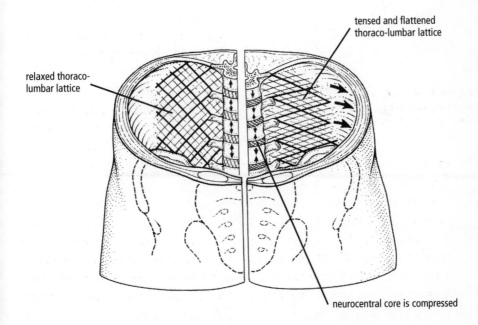

relaxed thoraco-lumbar lattice

tensed and flattened thoraco-lumbar lattice

neurocentral core is compressed

Figure 1.27 Transversus abdominus—a super-duper muscle-in-the-round—pulls the tummy in at the front and straightens the spine via the thoraco-lumbar fascia at the back.

invariably elicits pain from the problem part.

The breathing control of the thoraco-lumbar fascia also explains why we automatically hold our breath when we lift. The held breath and the clenched tummy recruit both muscle systems simultaneously, raising the tone in the thoraco-lumbar fascia. The lumbar segments are held doubly secure.

This is exactly what weight-lifters do. As they bend to grasp the bar they take a sharp breath in and hold it, sucking their tummy at the same time. Some professionals even wear a 'kidney belt' to reinforce the power of transversus abdominus, making it easier to generate the power to slot the lumbar vertebrae back on one another as the muscle pulls the spine straight.

2 The stiff spinal segment

This is the first stage in the breakdown of the spine, when one vertebra becomes stiffer than the rest, like a stiff link in a bicycle chain.

WHAT IS A STIFF SPINAL SEGMENT?

In the well-oiled spinal chain, a stiff spinal segment is a sluggish vertebra which participates less willingly than the others in overall spinal movement. More often than not the stiffer one causes no trouble; it just sits there being coaxed along by other more vigorous neighbours—and also being compensated for by them. When the spine performs its usual flourishing grandiose activity, they contribute a tiny bit more to make up for the stiff segment doing a little bit less.

Most spines have a patchy distribution of stiff links randomly spread throughout, from the base of the skull down to the sacrum. Some areas of the spine are naturally less mobile than others. The neck for example is more freewheeling in all its movements, while the low back is a much more fundamental pillar of support. In other parts of the spine, some movements are generous and others meagre. In the thoracic region, sideways bending is never very expansive because the ribs are in the way, but rotation or twist here is very free.

In the low back, all freedoms are kept to a minimum except forward bending. Most of the anatomical details of this part of the spine are designed to help it perform this single most important role. In a sense the main function of the low back is to make the skeleton bendable in the middle and therefore adjustable in height. It makes it possible to raise and lower your hands, eyes, ears and mouth by letting the upper 'thinking' part of your body get to the positions it needs to.

It is interesting that in the low back, the least mobile and most mobile lumbar segments are vertically adjacent. The fifth lumbar vertebra (L5) at the bottom of the spine, is the least mobile segment. Immediately on top is L4 which is the most mobile lumbar segment. Although it too can get stiff, it should come as no surprise then that L4 is the most likely lumbar segment to suffer from over-mobility problems (see Chapter 6, 'Segmental instability').

L5 on the other hand, is the most likely spinal segment to be too stiff.

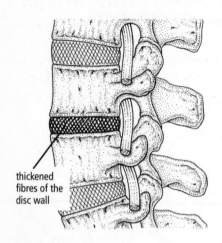

thickened
fibres of the
disc wall

Figure 2.1 The disc of a stiff spinal segment often looks like a narrowed 'washer' between its vertebrae.

The first cause of low back trouble

A chief factor which paves the way for stiffness of the low lumbar segments is the squashing pressure at the base of the spine. The discs between the lower vertebrae are compressed by being at the bottom of the stack. If they are squashed more than they are sucked apart there is a net loss of fluid from the discs as they gradually dry out. As they lose fluid they become stiffer, the lower ones faster than the upper ones, and the vertebrae sitting on top lose freedom to move. This manifests as a typical bruised feeling across the centre of the low back, known in the old days as lumbago.

A less mobile segment becomes an easy target for trauma because it cannot absorb shock as easily as the rest. Its vertebra cannot roll with the punches and is therefore susceptible to being knocked out of alignment. An ill-considered move can leave the problem vertebra locked and twisted on its axis, rather like a screw-top lid of a jar locking down when it is twisted home. If severe enough, the bump through the skin (which is the tail of the vertebra) will be visibly out of line with the rest. More commonly though, it manifests as a reluctance for the knob to be pushed transversely one way compared to the other. The pain from this sort of problem is usually felt on one side of the back only.

Protective muscle spasm

After injury, protective guarding by the muscles surrounding the injured segment keeps it out of action until the inflammation dies down. Usually this takes a day or so and then the muscles relax by degrees, letting in just enough movement to coax the injured fibres to heal. Tentatively at first and then with more gusto, they let the injured segment join in with the rest of the spine. All going well, movement introduced at just the right rate brings the injured segment back to full function and there is no legacy of pain. But if the injured link never gets going again properly, it will be an ongoing focus of future trouble.

Sometimes, overzealous muscle spasm can cause a stiff link in the spine, even though the original injury was minor. The vertical clench compresses the spine down its length, especially at the problem level. Over time, the tissues develop adaptive shortening across the interbody joint which is known as soft tissue contracture (like the children's fable where the changing wind fixes a grimace on the face). Thus one vertebra acts like a rusty link in the sleek spinal chain, clonking as the spine moves and sending out screeches of pain.

There can be a similar outcome if the muscle spasm remains self-fuelling, well after the initial cause has faded away. This is usually related to subliminal anxieties and a fear of moving the back, when it seems as if the muscles develop a mind of their own. They remain rigidly on guard (the muscles do not pulsate, which is a common misconception), restricting all spinal movement and making everything stiffer and more painful. The cycle is never easy to interrupt and in the self treatment section you will see how you may have to trick the muscles physiologically into switching off before progress can start.

Pain from simple segmental stiffness has no doubt been around since we evolved to stand upright. Using the hands to get all the vertebrae in line and equally mobile probably went on when we were cave dwellers in a way, believe it or not, which is still appropriate today. On the wall in my clinic I have a print of an ancient Egyptian text with diagrams of human spines being pushed around by the feet, a method I still use today.

However, this book is about self treatment and I will explain how doing a variety of exercises, using a block of wood, a tennis ball, or perhaps a convoluted rolling pin, can prise individual segments free using your own efforts. All that comes later. Meanwhile, back to the diagnosis.

CAUSES OF SEGMENTAL STIFFNESS

1. **The disc loses water and becomes thinner**
   - Gravity squeezes fluid from the discs
   - Poor movement prevents fluid replacement
   - The disc breaks down
2. **Other factors make it worse**
   - Sitting compresses the base of the spine
   - Abnormal postures increase neurocentral compression
   - Tummy weakness allows spine to 'sink'
   - Injury can rupture the cartilage plate between vertebra and disc

Gravity squeezes fluid from the discs

Several background factors make spinal segments susceptible to injury. The most fundamental is the incipient drying and thinning of the discs at the bottom of the stack because they carry the weight of the rest of the spine on top.

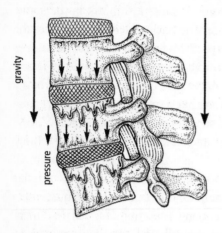

To tolerate this weight-bearing through a lifetime, the L5 disc starts off thicker than the rest. However constant downward pressure causes the lower discs to leach fluid and flatten, and radiographers commonly observe a loss of disc height at the bottom of the spine. It is very common for L5 to end up the thinnest disc in the spine.

Jogging is particularly damaging in that it forces fluid out of the lower discs. Marathon running can cause measurable shrinkage of the spine (of several centimetres). Faster running is better because one lands on the forefoot rather than the heel, which reduces impact. The greater effort and the forward stance also braces the tummy which lessens the ramming down effect on the base of the spine.

Figure 2.2 All discs lose fluid during upright hours, the lower ones faster than the upper ones.

Poor movement prevents fluid replacement

To some extent, discs hydrate themselves by using grand-scale spinal activity to pull the segments apart, thus creating a suction effect to entice fluids in from the neighbouring vertebral bodies. Unfortunately the relative stability of L5 equates to a lack of mobility, which makes it harder for this segment in particular to recoup lost fluids. As the most squashed disc, it is also the most disadvantaged; the trade-off between mobility and stability makes it harder for L5 to keep itself puffed up with fluid.

This is all the more so if the spine is less active for some reason. If you have pain, or fear movement, or you have faithfully followed instructions never to bend your spine, the lower discs flatten faster. Without sufficient bending and straightening of your back, the pressure changes within the discs are less adequate at shunting fluids in and out. Consequently, there is a steady squeezing dry of the low back, particularly the L5 disc, and its vertebra settles down lower on the sacral table.

To a degree, this happens to all the discs through the course of each day. The bearing down effect of gravity squeezes fluid from each one, from the base of the skull to the sacrum. This means we all go to bed appreciably shorter than when we got up. Overnight as our muscles relax and our spine stretches out along the mattress, our discs slowly swell. By morning we are tall again, our discs plumped up and primed, ready to take on another day.

Rejuvenation will be incomplete however, if we do not routinely bend and stretch with vigour throughout the daylight hours. With low activity levels our muscles and other soft tissues become less yielding and stretchable, which makes them less free to unravel so the body can unkink and 'grow' overnight. Thus our overall body stiffness increases compression of the discs. Because they are rarely put through their paces by day they are too stiff to let fluid seep in at night.

Movement is the life blood of the discs. In the past, studies have been conducted on patients confined to bed for non-back related problems. Measurement of their disc spaces before and after bed rest revealed that even healthy discs flatten with inactivity. How important it is that less healthy spines are made to move!

People who deliberately spare their backs by bending their knees instead, are actually doing harm. It starves the discs of drink. Certainly, if a weight is very heavy you should lift it like a weightlifter does, but for most daily travails—bending down to the bottom drawer, reaching up to the top cupboard—you must make your back do the work. *It is good for it.* If you persist with a straight back you will be bringing on your own demise; it makes your back stiffer, more fragile and more likely to give trouble.

You see this awkward bending with long-term back sufferers all the time— and they think they are doing what's best. As they bend over to wipe the table or tune the radio they keep their backs rigid and bend sideways in preference to going forward; otherwise they squat on their haunches with their spines ramrod straight. The often-cited reason for doing it this way is to reduce the pressure on the discs. And even this is wrong. It has been shown that the intradiscal pressure is just the same with bending (and lifting) whether the knees are bent or not.

Your extreme stiffness often makes you misread the cues; you are more likely to interpret bending as a no-go area if your back is painful. But be warned. Protecting your back in this way only makes things worse. It emphasises the use of the wrong muscles and makes the deep muscles of your spine and tummy so weak they cannot hold the segments together (see Chapters 4 and 6). Most importantly, it makes the problem levels vulnerable to shearing strains as the spine bends and lifts. One mishap when your back is working under duress can transform a benign correctable problem into a tragically incurable one.

The disc breaks down

As your back gets progressively less mobile the changes to the lower discs become irreversible. With the vertebrae pressed together the water content diminishes and the fibrous mesh of the disc wall becomes more fibrotic. The stiff wall imprisons the buoyant nucleus, like a child's flower press where four wing nuts in each corner screw down the top wooden plate, and the robust bouncing-back nucleus is kept penned inside, where it gradually gets more viscid (sludgy).

As the whole disc hardens it ceases to be a stretchable spinal connector. Commonly the bottom vertebra almost fuses itself to the sacrum, and a brittle junction comes into existence where the spine expects to move. You develop a stiff and vulnerable link, right where the spine should be uncomplainingly accommodating. You keep on demanding movement from a joint which cannot provide it and you keep hurting it. As a consequence the lower back becomes more painful with every move you make.

The adaptive shortening and stiffening of other ligaments which cross the intervertebral space make the changes to the disc more permanent. They peg down its mobility even more which greatly impairs the nutrition of the disc and makes the nucleus degrade further. As its molecular make-up alters, the nucleus loses its power to attract water and so it cannot keep itself puffed up under pressure. It fails to thrust the vertebrae apart to pre-tense the meshed wall and the disc collapses like a buckling wicker basket as weight bears down through it.

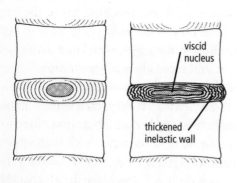

viscid
nucleus

thickened
inelastic wall

Figure 2.3 A healthy disc has a quivering up-thrust which defies gravity, whereas a degenerated one receives shock with a thud as it flattens out under pressure.

When as brittle as this, the poorly spring-loaded disc cannot ride out ripples passing through the spine. In effect the stiffer disc becomes a very 'knockable' link, sitting in a part of the spine where it unerringly gets knocked. It happens all the time: every time you rick your back and feel a glitch of pain, you have stressed the too-stiff link. As recent stiffness piles upon pre-existing stiffness the disc becomes a mere remnant of what it was. It becomes like a wedge of hard carpet between its two vertebrae instead of a vigorously tipping ball, springing them apart.

It is also difficult for a non-shock-absorbing disc to cope with bending and it is this action which converts a very stiff link into a stretched, tugged-apart one. As well as the inertness of the disc, the tiny muscles controlling the stiff segment atrophy because they have so little to do. This combination makes the brittle link even more vulnerable to trauma, and can be the first stage in the development of spinal instability.

The purpose of self treatment is to get this stiff link more mobile so it is no longer vulnerable, and then to strengthen the weak link so it can fend off trouble in future.

Sitting compresses the base of the spine

The pressure inside the discs is higher with sitting than standing or lying. The sacral table rams up under the descending spine and the base is pinched in the middle as if caught in a vertical vice. Over time, fluid leaks out of the discs (they lose approximately 10 per cent of their total fluid) and the stacked bony segments settle together, becoming a semi-rigid tubular mass. Most of the fluid escapes within the first hour or two of sitting, but the discs keep squeezing drier the longer they stay compressed. People who sit for long hours to work usually feel cast in the back when they get up. It can take several minutes before the base of the spine drops down and movement gets easier. If long hours of sitting are combined with low levels of activity the lowest discs never properly reflate.

The discs puff up again with fluid faster than they expel it. This is partly due to concentration of electrolytes in the nuclear gel which drags in water under osmotic pressure, but also through the suction effect of the spine elongating when unweighted. The discs puff up more quickly if you lie on your back and bring your knees to your chest which is why this simple action is such an important part of self treatment. Bouncing your knees to chest and squatting exercises through the day help counteract the fluid loss from the discs, mainly by hinging open the *back* of your spine.

On the other hand, using a BackBlock opens the *front* of your spine. It passively hyper-extends (over arches) your spine which not only opens the front of the discs and drags fluid in but also reverses the slumped posture of sitting. As part of your self treatment program, you should use the Block every day. I promise you will get addicted to the sensation of the segments pulling apart, when you can almost feel the flattened mesh walls of the discs being tugged up and water being dragged in from the vertebral bodies through the sieve-like vertebral end-plates.

Many hours of sitting can also cause adaptive shortening of other structures around the low back which makes resuming a normal posture even more difficult. For example, the hip flexor muscles at the front of your hips are very powerful and tighten quickly when they spend long periods puckered in a shortened state. Their tethering causes a sense of tightness across the front of the hips and down the thighs which makes it difficult to stand up straight.

In the long term this tightness has adverse consequences because it causes the front of the pelvis to tilt down at the front, which throws the spine out of balance and creates a typical 'bottom out' appearance. Tight hip flexors also make you take much shorter steps because the legs cannot angle back properly at the hips. Again this is bad for the back because in making a decent stride, the spine must twist left and right to compensate for the poor hip mobility.

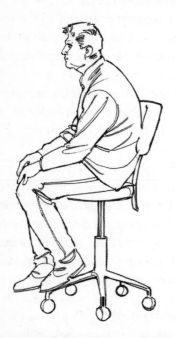

Figure 2.4 Slumped sitting is one of the chief compressors of the spine and a BackBlock is the best way to pull it out.

If the sitting posture is especially slumped it causes adaptive contracture of the anterior longitudinal ligament which runs down the front of the vertebral bodies like a long elastic tape. In healthy circumstances its role is to limit the backward arching movement of the spine, but when it adaptively shortens it tethers the spine over in a hoop at the front, like an over-tight bowstring. People are often aware of their worsening posture, and feel they are being kept stooped, as if their shirt is tucked too tightly into their waist band.

Using the BackBlock is the natural antidote for sitting. It helps undo all the problems acquired by hours spent crimped at the hips and knees with the shoulders curled forward over the task at hand. It opens out the bowed-over spine and chest, it pushes in the bottom and stretches out the front of the hips as the legs drop down to the floor. But most importantly, it decompresses the spine by pulling up the bunched down disc walls and sucking in fluid.

Bear in mind that sitting, or parking our pelvis on a chair, is a recent and fairly unnatural phenomenon. Many indigenous people still squat rather than use high-backed support. Even though their day may involve running or carrying heavy loads, both of which compress the base of the spine, they can easily disimpact it again come nightfall by squatting to prepare food and eat. You would never see a Masai warrior slumped on a sofa. Frequent squatting exercises form a large part of the self treatment program.

Most sedentary jobs bring on a degree of segmental stiffness of the low back. Sitting hunched and scrunched on a chair—often with the legs crossed and the telephone glued to the ear—stiffens the whole body and dries out the base of the spine. Computer operators, machinists, or anybody who sits at a bench or desk working all day, are particularly susceptible. As the hours mount up, they get stiffer more quickly each time they sit, and take longer to straighten after getting up; a persistent broad band of immobility across the base of the spine eventually becomes overt trouble.

Long-distance drivers and taxi drivers also have a high incidence of back trouble. Apart from the sitting, the continuous vibration of the vehicle causes a greater loss of fluid from the lower discs. Truck drivers are even more prone to back trouble if the cabin is high up and they have to jump a long way to the ground. The impact is particularly jarring when the spine is already compressed. Matters are made worse if they have to push heavy objects around in preparation for lifting on and off the tray.

Abnormal postures increase neurocentral compression

Deviant spinal alignment can be a potent cause of segmental stiffening. Anomalies can stem from poor postural habits, just as much as from congenital curvatures like spinal scoliosis.

As a rule, spinal segments stiffen more readily in zones where the spine's function alters; where it changes from neck to thorax to low back. These are called the transition zones and they correspond to where 'S' curves (viewed sideways on) change direction. Hence, the common trouble spots in the spine are the lumbo-sacral level (where the spine joins the fixed pelvis), the thoraco-lumbar level (where the thorax becomes the lower back), the cervico-thoracic level (where the neck joins the thorax) and the atlanto-occipital joint (where the neck joins the base of the skull).

A rounded (kyphotic) low back

All transition zones give greater trouble if the regular 'S' bend of the spine deviates too far from normal. However, a fixed kyphotic low back (rounded into a hump instead of a hollow) is particularly troublesome for the neurocentral core because the facet joints at the back take no weight at all. Many spinal levels develop segmental stiffness because of unremitting compression and difficulty in absorbing shock.

A fixed kyphosis creates a poorer exchange of fluids through the lower discs. As the spine pile-drives down into itself, there is a less than vigorous fluid movement because the natural bowing sink and spring does not exist. At the time it needs it most, the excessively jarred lower back has to make do with reduced nutrition to carry out vital running repairs. This only heightens the natural attrition of weight-bearing activity and the back wears out faster.

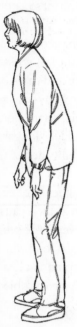

Running with a humped low back is an exceptional hazard. The spine cannot bow gracefully into a shock-receiving hollow like a hoop bending as it receives impact, and all the shock is taken up through the neurocentral core. As your weight descends earthwards through the body, the lumbar segments cannot squelch forward on their discs to dissipate the downward forces. Apart from the incessant jarring which affects the whole frame, there is also no corresponding uplift to spring the spine skywards which can pull up the disc walls. Even walking can be juddering instead of feline and youthful, with the head no longer tracing an imaginary wavy line along through the air as the spine bounces along with every step.

Figure 2.5 A permanently stooped low back causes too much weight to pass down through the neurocentral core.

Even the most youthful spines collapse into a 'C' shape when sitting, but it is better if they keep a proper lordosis. This applies even more when sitting in a vehicle when the added vibration causes greater fluid loss. Accordingly, car seats should have a firm and pronounced upholstered bulge filling out the entire lumbar hollow (to the extent that it feels too much when you first sit down) and the seat should not be tipped down at the back which throws you into slumped sitting on the neurocentral core.

Incidentally, the correct horse riding attitude is almost the perfect posture for the back to disperse weight. Providing the stirrups are the right length, the low back assumes the optimum alignment to ride out shock and balance the upper body over the pelvis.

There is another ill effect of lumbar kyphosis. It means that the weight of the upper body is carried too far forward, in front of the line of gravity; the spine cannot stack itself with minimumal effort, which causes a 'turning moment' (a tendency for the upper spine to move forward) around the thoraco-lumbar junction. With the shoulders stooped, the lumbar segments slide forward, jamming the spine at mid-lumbar level. A lumbar kyphosis creates a similar tendency for the whole body to tip forward on the pelvis, also contributing to the typical 'bottom out' appearance.

This is a great source of strain. Pain can emanate from two sites—the bottom and top ends of the lumbar spine—at the same time. Upper lumbar problems often refer pain down lower in the back over the lumbo-sacral junction. When isolating your problem levels it is important not to assume that all your trouble is coming from L5, where the pain is. Both levels must be dealt with if you are to get better.

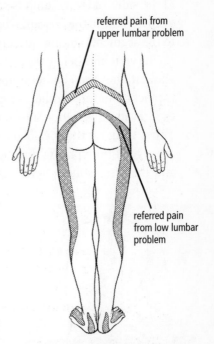

Figure 2.6 Segments in both the upper and lower lumbar spine can refer pain to a similar area across the top of the buttocks.

A sideways twisted (scoliotic) spine

Spinal scoliosis is a lateral 'S' shaped twist through the spine which is obvious when viewed from behind. It can be a congenital abnormality or caused by a shorter leg. If the scoliotic curves are relatively stable and do not involve rotation of the vertebrae, the pathology will limit itself to segmental jamming. If however the spine twists as well as deviates laterally, the disorder will include facet joint trouble (see Chapter 3). The facets become chronically inflamed in their taxing role of locking the spinal segments together to prevent them toppling off one other.

With scoliosis the curvature usually consists of a primary curve in the lower back and a secondary curve higher up the spine. The upper curve develops to compensate for the lower one, throwing the spine back across the central line so the head sits squarely on the shoulders at the top of the column, allowing the eyes to focus.

When one leg is shorter, the spine usually twists one way then the other, compensating in a fairly predictable way. For example, if your right leg is shorter and your pelvis dips to the right, your spine leans initially to the right, making a lateral sweeping curve, convex to the right. Higher up your spine there will be another lesser curve convex to the left, to tip the spine back the other way.

Lateral curves in the spine lead to trouble because the ligamentous shoring of the sides of the column is so weak. Unlike the various structures which keep it stable in the forwards–backwards direction, there is little impediment to the segments sliding sideways off one another except the disc wall itself.

The vertebrae below the apex of the curve tend to slide one way, and those above it, the other. Rather unfortunately, the vertebra at the peak of the apex is pinched in the middle, compressing its intervertebral disc beneath it. As the travelling vertebrae move off-centre their discs are dragged sideways. Thus the disc at the apex of the curve is flattened and the neighbouring ones are tugged in opposing directions. In all cases, the disc walls bunch down and the discs stiffen. Several contiguous discs end up thinner with their

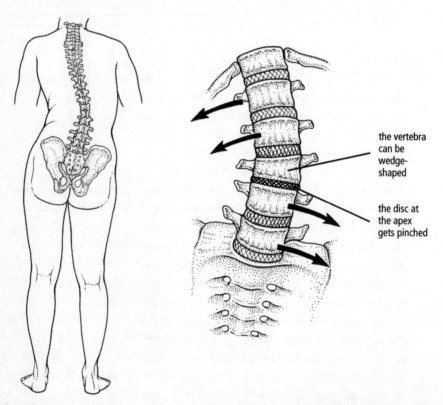

the vertebra can be wedge-shaped

the disc at the apex gets pinched

Figure 2.7 When viewed from behind, scoliosis appears as a lateral 'S' shaped bend through the spine.

Figure 2.8 Due to poor lateral shoring of the spine, scoliotic segments tend to creep sideways in one direction below a curve's apex, and the other way above.

vertebrae sluggish—which explains why scoliotic spines can be so worrying, with such a diffuse spread of pain.

The pain from the jammed apical segments is always the greatest. There may be several of them, depending how many times the spine twists back and forth as it goes up. These focal points account for the wide variety of symptoms which go with scoliosis. There can be pain in the neck (sometimes including headaches), in the shoulder blade area (sometimes down the arm), pain in the back beside the waist (sometimes referred to the groin), and pain in the low back (sometimes referred into the buttock or down the leg). With so much pain at once, mild scoliotic patients in particular are rarely taken seriously and often wrongly dismissed as malingerers.

Symptoms from exaggerated spinal curves (lordotic and kyphotic low backs) usually emerge during the third decade of life as the internal make-up of the tissues changes and they become more fibrous. Pain from scoliosis, on the other hand, can come on as early as nine or ten years old and be with you for life, getting progressively worse, unless you do something about it.

Tummy weakness allows the spine to 'sink'

Although a hard, statically contracted tummy plays a critical role as a retaining wall when the spine bends, it also does important things just as you sit there. A strong co-contraction with the back muscles buoys the spine up and stops the segments telescoping down into the pelvis and compressing the discs.

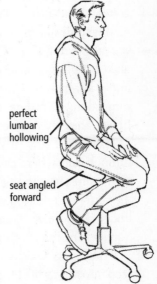

perfect lumbar hollowing

seat angled forward

When the abdominal retaining wall is weak, it cannot generate enough upthrust on the lumbar segments to offset the downward forces. The low intra-abdominal pressure cannot lift the spine and interrupt the bearing down pressures on the base. As the girth expands with sitting and the belly falls forward over the belt like a bag of chaff, the abdominal contents spill forward, dragging the spine downwards. As the multi-segmented column ploughs down ever more firmly onto the sacrum, it increases the pressure on the lower discs.

By moving forward onto the front of the seat incidentally, the abdominal wall works more dynamically and gives better support. You can see this for yourself. If you sit slumped on a sofa

Figure 2.9 The kneeling chair creates an 'almost perfect' sitting posture.

your tummy balloons forward, flaccid and inert. If you sit up free of back support you feel the internal corsetry of your tummy reefing in the retaining wall and making a firm, flexible cylinder. It also makes the top of your spine better balanced and free-wheeling to work more efficiently over its base.

The best sitting arrangement at a desk is a kneeling chair. Its seat is inclined forward a few degrees which promotes optimal hollowing of the lumbar spine instead of a slumped 'C'. Some weight taken through the knees and lower legs on the upholstered cushion minimises that taken through the lower back. But even though it is ingenious, this chair should be used with caution if you have knee or ankle problems, or if your low back already has too much lumbar arch.

It is worth noting that carrying loads balanced on the head—another time honoured custom of less developed societies—invokes a superb dynamic response from the tummy muscles. Automatically they pull in and brace, converting the lower abdomen into a taut, supportive cylinder. The raised pressure within the abdominal cavity creates extra lift for the spine and safeguards the lower segments from excessive compression. We might do well to copy this way of carrying.

Injury can rupture the cartilage plate between vertebra and disc

Unlike the hard cortical bone making up the sides of the vertebrae, the vertebral end-plates of the top and bottom are a thin cartilaginous interface. As the spine alternately compresses and off-loads like a concertina during weight-bearing activity, the trapped internal pressure of the discs naturally makes the end-plates belly outwards with the force, like wind billowing up under a tarpaulin. This gives us a lovely buoyant spring in our step as we romp along a pavement, but it also illustrates how weak the end-plates are. In fact, they are the weakest component part of the spine.

There are many tiny holes in the end-plates where blood vessels come through and where cavities in the honeycomb bone beyond the cartilage abut against it. Although they allow the diffusion of fluids into the discs from the vertebral bodies they are pinpoints of weakness and can easily perforate under pressure. As a reverberating shock passes up through the central core, a small vent can rupture through the fibro-cartilage interface.

If the disc is healthy, the tiny fracture can allow blood from the vertebra to seep into the sterile bloodless outer environs of the disc. In a process similar to a cold abscess, a low grade 'discitis' (or inflammatory reaction) may set up in the disc as it reacts to the blood.

The process may be completely painless, because it is contained within the insensitive interior part of the disc, but usually the segment stiffens afterwards. It turns into a fibrous 'washer' which pads out the interspace and gives the disc some bulk. But thereafter the fibrosed mass can only operate as a primitive sort of spacer. It can separate the vertebrae well enough but it has none of the high performance, high tensile spinal connector properties which make a healthy one so brilliant at what it does.

There are many ways you can puncture a vent in the bone, but the most common is stepping off a wall while carrying a heavy weight (particularly on your shoulder) or falling down hard on your bottom (especially if you were expecting a chair to be there). You may also do it wrenching up a sash window which is stuck, or standing up suddenly and hitting your head on an overhead beam (although this is more likely to injure the thoracic part of the spine).

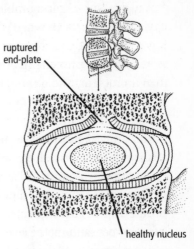

ruptured end-plate

healthy nucleus

Figure 2.10 It is relatively easy to punch a tiny hole through the vertebral end-plate.

Dramatic as the original trauma may be at the time, it rarely causes severe pain. It jars the spine but discomfort is usually short-lived. Your back may feel stiff and sore for a few days, possibly with some leg pain from the trauma to the facets. However, you are often aware, in a vague sort of way, that your back is never quite the same again. The injury is often the fast track route to developing a stiff spinal segment, as the disc hardens and narrows and settles into an inert space-filling role.

The process is even less painful when it happens higher up the spine. Often you are unaware of anything wrong until X-rays reveal a typical tear-drop anomaly in the main body of a vertebra called a Schmorl's node. But lower down the spine the higher stresses can cause the sick disc to degenerate much faster, sometimes resulting in the entirely different symptoms of segmental instability (see Chapter 6).

THE WAY THIS BACK BEHAVES

There is a world of difference between the acute and chronic forms of the stiff spinal segment. Strange to say, the more advanced pathologies are often less painful. This is because the segment is so stiff it is almost fused, and where there is little movement there is little pain.

The sub-clinical phase

In its sub-clinical form this back is hardly a problem. It may be stiff after a long car trip or sleeping in a different bed, but it is never painful. There may be a vague awareness that something is not right with your back, but for years it may come to nothing more than this.

A typical sub-clinical problem is the 'jumpy legs' syndrome, which feels as if two live wires touch when you sit for too long. A lesser form of the affliction is not being able to keep your legs still when sitting, usually combined with a dull sense of pressure in your back. Both conditions are more a nuisance than a problem, and although there is never any pain, it is unnerving and indicates a degree of compression of the spine which is an ill omen for the future.

Sub-clinical disorders wait in the wings to cause trouble. The causing mishap is often trivial, yet brings about an extraordinary pain response. People are often perplexed at how their back became painful so quickly with so little provocation. But they actually had it coming; their back was silently protecting a rusty level and adjusting for its lack of mobility by over-compensating at the levels above and below. For some reason, the ricking incident bypasses all the usual defences, and unavoidably targets the semi-rigid link.

The acute phase

There is no greater backpain than acute inflammation of a spinal segment. It causes an intense smarting, aching soreness right across the centre of the

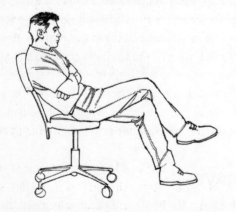
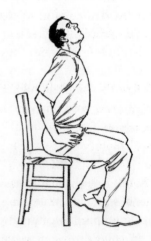

Figure 2.11 With acute segmental stiffness, the spine does not like being 'sat on'—you either lie back on a slung-out spine or over-arch to relieve the pressure.

back which is often too tender to touch. It is often described as screamingly painful with a hot throbbing sensation under the skin, like a boil about to burst. (When this bad it is common to suspect you have cancer.) If the vertebra is locked one way, twisted on its axis, the pain will still be central but focused to one side as well.

At the height of an acute condition your back feels as fragile as a Dresden doll. Jarring it can be so painful it almost makes you sick. Even deviating in your path to avoid a collision on the footpath can make you so weak you almost crumple at the knees. Someone brushing past behind can make you flinch, and automatically move out of the way. Staying upright may be nearly impossible, although pressing the flat of your back into the wall can give you relief. Cooking the dinner can be a panicky race against time, until the pain makes you lie down.

Sitting is uncomfortable and your spine does not like being compressed. You constantly shift positions from slumping deeply and resting on the low slung-out back (to take the pressure off the neurocentral core) to perching forward and making it over-arch (so the facets take more weight). Either way, your back is uncomfortable again within moments. Even lying down can be painful because your back feels too tender to take the pressure. The locked vertebra seem pushed up by the muscles, as if you are lying on a stone.

Acute palpation

When I use my hands to palpate, the vertebra can be highly sensitive to light pressure but surprisingly less so to deep. En masse, the vertebrae feel bunched together, like a row of beads threaded too tightly on elastic. Sometimes the segments feel hard to depress like piano keys where the spring underneath is too stiff. Often the surrounding tissues have a puffy, water-logged feel with a deep inflammatory heat smouldering up from below.

What causes the acute pain?

With acute segmental stiffness there are multifarious reasons for the pain and there is plenty of it.

The injury which first hurts your back can be likened to a ligament strain of the disc. It is similar to spraining an ankle though on a smaller scale. Chemical toxins are released when the fibres are damaged which irritate 'nociceptors' or free nerve endings in the disc wall. Messages are relayed to the brain from the injured part which are interpreted as pain.

Having said this, the disc is poorly sensitive to pain. Only the outer layers of its wall have a nerve supply which makes it unlikely to bring about intense pain on its own. This rather points to the cramp of local muscles in spasm and the accumulation of waste products around the injury as other sources of pain.

Although the muscle spasm is protective it can be too unrelenting. Unabated, it physically jams the segments together and increases the pain coming from the sore interbody joint. Mechanical receptors with bulbous or globular nerve endings in the disc wall are stimulated by the excessive compression. These are situated between the fibres and are sensitive to physical distortion. They are flattened when the disc is flattened and this too is perceived as pain. Sometimes this stimulates more protective reaction from the muscles and the painful cycle intensifies.

Probably most of the pain comes from the intense vascular engorgement around the injured part when the muscles prevent free movement. The disc stays bloated from compression and the circulation of blood becomes sluggish because there is no pumping action from free movement to sluice it on. Pain comes from the physical engorgement of the neighbouring pain-sensitive structures and also from the rising concentration of waste products in the stale blood.

This engorgement is a potent source of discomfort. It accounts for the steadily increasing pain, several hours after injury, just like when you twist an ankle. There is a wrench of pain when the mishap first happens which then passes off, but several hours later the pain worsens. As the joint gets stiffer and more tense with swelling, there is a frightening inexorability about the way the pain gets worse.

The sub-acute phase

In this phase, the discomfort from the low back is more bearable. The lumbar spine feels permanently clenched, with peaks of stinging pain or twinges whenever it gets tired. It suddenly gets uncomfortable being in one position for too long and is only relieved by moving about. Rubbing with the flat of the hand is a relief, although direct pressure on the vertebra feels tender, as if the bone itself is bruised. The aching stiffness can be relieved by heat, sometimes so hot it works like a counter-irritant. (Using a hot water bottle is common but often leaves a mottled discolouration of the skin which takes years to fade.)

Movement is painful because the muscles are tight and the back fails to let go as you try to push through their clench. Standing becomes more painful as the spine becomes more cast. It worsens into brittle impaction if you stay there and then it hurts to sit down. The spine cannot pull its segments apart to get itself rounded, and folding up to get into the car after a cocktail party for example, can be excruciating.

From the sub-acute phase, the problem can pitch back into acute flare-ups when the jammed link is disturbed or it can become more subdued and move into the chronic phase. It typically see-saws between the two with painful spates and remissions, and shorter respites in between. At this stage, avoiding hurting your back can become life's obsession. You take the long way round doing everything, just to avoid setting it off, and often the whole family must come to terms with accommodating your back.

Sub-acute palpation

When I palpate with my hands the segments have usually lost their bunched together feel, but there will be a tubular rigidity across a local section of the neurocentral core. The spine feels brittle, as if the cotton reels are welded together and the surrounding tissues may have the rubbery feel of longstanding inflammation. With the flat of my hand I feel the drag of moisture on the skin which indicates a deep seated, low grade inflammation. After manually mobilising the vertebrae the skin often flushes up red with the blood rushing to the surface. (The degree of redness gives some indication of the degree of inflammation.)

The chronic phase

The chronic phase of segmental stiffness makes you feel years older than you are. Rather than frank pain you have a deep, aching, armour-plated stiffness across your low back. Arching backwards gives relief, but bending forward is always awkward and stiff; your back feels so rigid you sense you shouldn't do it. It is difficult drying your toes and putting your socks on in the morning but activity gets easier as the day goes on. You feel ancient getting out of a chair or car and you often have to winch yourself straight before moving off.

Chronic palpation

Delving around in a spine like this, it seems the fire has gone out leaving only the cold embers. There is no soupy inflammatory feel of the tissues because they are so inert and lacking in juice they barely react. The vertebral column feels like a semi-rigid mass with thickened bars of bone across the segmental junctions. Often the bone of the vertebrae feels enlarged, like barnacles encrusted to an anchor chain, and the segments have a rock-hard blocking resistance to passive gliding pressures from me.

What causes the chronic pain?

When a stiff spinal segment passes from its acute to chronic phase the pain comes about for different reasons.

During the course of everyday activity most of the weight through the segment is taken by the disc wall. This causes the wall to flatten, and the bulbous mechanical receptors hidden between the fibres are stimulated. If fibres are pulverised and broken by excessive compression the chemical receptors will be activated by the toxins of injury. Thus the brain receives two different pain messages.

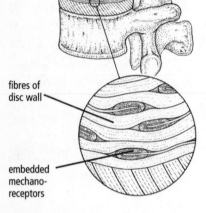

fibres of disc wall

embedded mechano-receptors

Figure 2.12 Bulbous mechano-receptors in the disc wall pick up both compression and tension of the wall fibres.

Pain can also be provoked by the stiff disc wall being stretched. When the disc is inelastic and not free to pull apart with the other segments, the mechano-receptors pick up the unhealthy lack of give in the fibres and interprets it as pain. If fibres are broken through being stretched beyond their limit, the chemo-receptors pick up the toxins released by the injured tissue.

Pain from tissue tightness can also be registered in the other ligaments which help the disc hold the vertebral space together, in particular the posterior longitudinal ligament. As the problem disc drops in height during the degenerative process there is adaptive shortening of the ligament across the interspace.

The posterior longitudinal ligament has a highly sophisticated nerve supply, and once a tight band develops the ligament will register pain—just like the disc only more so—when provoked by stretch. Because it runs right down the back of the vertebral bodies, its tightness makes bending forward particularly painful.

WHAT YOU CAN DO ABOUT IT

Aims of self treatment for segmental stiffness

No matter what the phase, the overriding mission with segmental stiffness is to reduce the compression of your basal spinal segments. This is much more straightforward with the chronic condition because your back is barely sore. It is achey and bone-deep stiff and although exercising may stir it up, the benefits are immediately apparent. Loosening the segments is achieved by using the BackBlock and doing squatting exercises, but then it is important to immediately make use of the newfound freedom to make it permanent.

When the back is acutely inflamed, muscle spasm is the wild card which complicates everything. Although its role is ultimately protective, much of the overall pain picture can be attributed to it locking up the spine and holding it too rigidly. Not only does this compress the segments more, it causes more pain from the muscle clench itself. Both factors make your back screamingly painful and also extremely unpredictable from one moment to the next.

Getting rid of the muscle spasm is the first priority, although all the techniques to do this help loosen the segments as well. Spasm in the muscle is reduced by stretching it through bouncing the knees to the chest, breaking up the brittle castness of the segments by rolling back and forth over the low back, and 'switching off' the back muscles by strengthening their opposite number (the tummy muscles) through making the tummy work hard during curl ups.

ATTENTION: Bending and touching your toes has long been held by conventional wisdom to be dangerous. However, I believe it is crucial for your recovery. Although it may hurt initially, keep your tummy braced and don't turn back!

A typical treatment for acute segmental stiffness

(See Chapter 7 for descriptions of all exercises and the correct way to do them.)

Purpose: Relieve muscle spasm, disperse inflammation

Rocking knees to the chest (60 seconds)

Rest (with knees bent for 30 seconds)

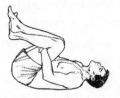

Rocking knees to the chest

Rest

Rocking knees to the chest

Curl ups (five times)

Rest

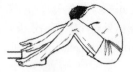

Rocking knees to the chest

Curl ups

Rest

Rocking knees to the chest

Curl ups

Rest

Rocking knees to the chest

Curl ups

Rest

Rest in bed and use medication of NSAIDS (anti-inflammatories), painkillers and muscle relaxants as directed by your doctor. Repeat exercises in bed every two hours.

For how long? This phase usually lasts anything from two or three days to a week. You can advance to the next treatment stage when it is easier to sit up and turn over in bed. Remember, fear holds you back. Relax in bed and stay floppy. If you jar your back, relieve the pain by rocking your knees to your chest and resting with your lower legs supported on pillows. Try to relax and not think about the pain.

A typical treatment for sub-acute segmental stiffness

Purpose: Stretch muscle spasm, disperse inflammation, tummy muscle activity to switch off the muscle spasm

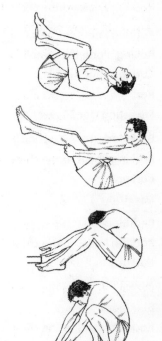

Rocking knees to chest (for 60 seconds)
Rolling along spine (for 15–30 seconds)
Curl ups (five times)
Rest
___

Rocking knees to the chest
Rolling along spine
Curl ups
Rest
___

Rocking knees to the chest
Rolling along spine
Curl ups
Rest
___

Squatting (for 30 seconds)
Curl ups
___

Squatting
Curl ups
___

Medication of painkillers and NSAIDS only. Two 20 minute rest periods each day. Repeat regimen on a folded towel on carpeted floor three times daily.

For how long? You may progress through this period in ten days to two weeks. It cannot be hurried and you need regular rest periods between exercises. Progress to the next regimen when the pain is intermittent and bending less painful.

A typical treatment for chronic segmental stiffness

Purpose: Reduce general stiffness by decompressing front and back of spine, strengthen tummy

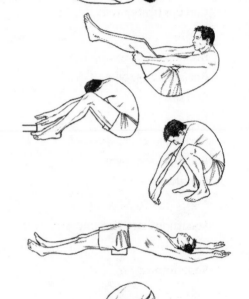

Rocking knees to chest (for 60 seconds)

Rolling along the spine (15–30 seconds)

Curl ups (five times)

Rest

Squatting (for 30 seconds)

––––––

BackBlock (for 60 seconds)

Rocking knees to the chest

Curl ups

Squatting

––––––

BackBlock

Rocking knees to the chest

Curl ups

Squatting

––––––

BackBlock

Rocking knees to the chest

Curl ups

Squatting

––––––

Toe touches (down and up three times)

––––––

Repeat program every evening before going to bed. Continue NSAIDS if back is too sore to exercise.

For how long? This phase may continue for several weeks but is prone to relapse if you do too much. Always sprinkle your day with toe touches, perhaps one or two per hour and always squat after lengthy periods of sitting. If soreness is uncontrollable, stop BackBlock (only) and revert to sub-acute regimen for two or three days.

A typical treatment for sub-chronic segmental stiffness

Purpose: Decompress spine front and back, strengthen tummy, restore trunk control

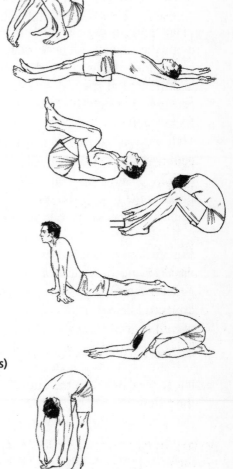

Squatting
BackBlock
Rocking knees to the chest
Curl ups (15 times)
___

Squatting
BackBlock
Rocking knees to the chest
Curl ups
___

Squatting
BackBlock
Rocking knees to the chest
Curl ups
___

Cobra (for 10 seconds)
Pose of the child (for 10 seconds)
___

Cobra
Pose of the child
___

Cobra
Pose of the child
___

Toe touches (down and up three times)
Squatting
___

Toe touches
Squatting
___

Repeat every evening before going to bed.

For how long? This regimen continues indefinitely. Continue daily with toe touching whenever you feel your back getting stiff, and always squat briefly after sitting. If there is a flare-up you should revert to the sub-acute regimen for two to three days, resuming the BackBlock, the Cobra and Pose of the Child as the pain fades.

A CASE HISTORY OF A STIFF SPINAL SEGMENT

Frances is a 45-year-old mother of two who had been in pain on and off for the past 14 years since the birth of her first child. She complained of chronic pain and stiffness straight across the low back in a broad spread just above the line of both lumbar dimples. It was uncomfortable sitting but worse getting up from a chair. Any sudden, unguarded movement would give a severe shaft of pain through the back and leave her back sore for several weeks.

Over the past two years it had been getting worse and now most activities in her daily life hurt. Her problems were compounded by days spent sitting doing the accounts for her husband's restaurant. She was unusually tall with an unathletic build, although not overweight. Her tummy was weak and she had the typical stooped posture of slightly rounded shoulders and lower back which meant she collapsed down into her pelvis rather than bearing herself aloft.

In my waiting room when I first saw her, I noticed she had difficulty getting out of a chair. She used both arm rests to haul herself forward and then by pushing up with both hands, she propelled her pelvis forward to position the base of the spine under the rest of her spine. In this way she could avoid bending while getting up from the seat.

Bending was Frances's greatest weakness. When I asked her to touch her toes she looked aghast. She felt vulnerable because it was a movement she usually avoided. Because of this, the muscles held so tightly she could barely go more than 15 or 20 degrees. The muscles beside the spine stood up like cables and slewed her off-centre, making her low back arch awkwardly instead of curling over. At the same time she had an unpleasant sensation of pain and tension covering the whole lumbar area.

It was even difficult getting her to lie prone on the treatment couch. She felt so weak through the midriff that she could not move herself up over the pillow. She had to get up on her hands and knees and move forward up the couch and then lie down in the right position. She could not shimmy herself up the couch with a wriggling action of her spine; it was too weak. Once in position, kneeling over the pillow, she had to take it slowly to lower her pelvis down flat. This showed that she was significantly disabled.

All became obvious when I palpated her spine. L5 was so immobile to forward gliding pressures that it felt almost welded to the sacrum. It was acutely tender to touch with the typical bruised bone feel but quite quickly the superficial brittleness yielded and it began to move.

Unusually for a condition this irritable, the tissues around the L5 segment did not exhibit the usual sort of soupy feel of longstanding inflammation, and this boded well for her future. The stiff L5 segment had a hard crisp feel which I knew from experience would respond well to mobilisation with minimal complications from treatment soreness. Frances was an ideal candidate to move along quickly.

My conclusions were that Frances's problem was a good example of a severely impacted L5 segment. (Her X-rays confirmed this by revealing the L5–S1 disc interspace reduced by half, with a bony spur at the front of the vertebral body.) A lesser problem but something which would need treatment later was a stiff L4 with its backward projecting spinous process swung across to the left.

Significantly though, I felt Frances was at the point of getting much worse. She demonstrated many signs of incipient instability (see Chapter 6) and the way she got out of the chair on first sight was ample evidence of this. She also showed marked imbalance of the muscles which control the spine and this is why she felt so insecure bending over. She exhibited the classic picture of a chronically bad back when the deep muscles of the spine automatically inhibit and leave the spine stiff and vulnerable on going over.

Typically, her lower tummy was very weak and she was unable to pull it in to actively brace the spine as she went over—a characteristic of transversus abdominus weakness. The intrinsic muscles at the back of her spine were also weak as evidenced by her inability to swell the lower back out and make it hump as she went forward. This is why the strong cable-like muscles beside the spine were working in overdrive and she could not curl over.

The dynamics of her muscular control were so discordant I felt she was indeed very close to developing instability (probably at the L5 level). She was stiff as a board at both bottom two levels but there was also a hollowed out empty feel around each segment, indicating wasting of the spinal intrinsic muscles there. This means she had been making do with the long superficial muscles holding her spine as best they could, in the typical clumsy guy rope way, similar to stabilising a tent pole.

In the way the base of a tent pole can flick across the ground if the tension of its guy ropes is too great, the base of Frances's spine was in danger of shifting (forward) as she bent. Intuitively she seemed to sense this danger and deliberately chose not to do it. Although she was getting weaker and more discommoded in her daily life, this seemed the lesser of two evils.

Apart from getting rid of her day-to-day pain, a seeming contradiction of her condition would have to be addressed if Frances was to get completely better: the stiff weak links in her spine had to be un-stiffened but at the same time, they had to acquire some strength.

First treatment

Because it was so difficult for Frances to lift her spine and move about (lifting her leg into the car was one of her most difficult tasks) I went straight to assisted curl ups exercise to restore strength to her tummy before attempting to mobilise the stiff segment. (If I were to treat her from the start in the prone position I know I would have great difficulty getting her up again which would have frightened her.)

Many curl ups were done in the proper way with the knees bent and me sitting on her feet and using my hands to help pull her up. Even lifting her head hurt at the start, which is commonly the case. So I helped her coming up but lessened my grip for her return journey to the couch. She was able to do this better, recruiting the lower abdominals group (transversus abdominus) which were so obviously weak. As she went down I let go more and more, so she controlled most of the action herself.

Although there is a lot of debate about sit-ups, I prefer them to be done as a full curling-up action because they achieve several things at once. Apart from providing much needed strength for Frances's weak lower abdomen, I needed them to automatically switch off the back muscles which had been in such spasm. Full range curling-up sit-ups also help mobilise the L4 and L5 segments by pressing over them (along with the others) during the rolling up and down action.

At first, the curl ups were not easy and caused a sharp pain when Frances was halfway up. This made her deviate to one side to go around the pain with an awkward slewing action. She also attempted to pull herself up with her spine straight rather than segmentally curling, which I did not like, and the effort appeared superhuman (she was crushing my hands in hers).

After the first few curl ups she was able to do them better with a proper curling action, and as she did so, the pinching pain in her back eased. After about ten of them I let her relax and asked her to gently oscillate her knees to her chest before repeating each batch several more times. (I told her I fully expected her tummy to feel strained in the next few days and that all going well, it should even hurt to laugh.)

I then got her up and turned her over onto her stomach and was pleased to note that she got up from the counch a shade more easily.

With Frances in the prone position, I then mobilised her jammed L5. Although it took some five minutes of gentle mobilising with the thumbs, the lessening of pain on my pressure eventually caught up with the easing of segmental movement. I did not continue longer because I wanted to avoid her getting cast on her tummy when trying to get up. As it was, it was quite difficult getting her up. I had to ask her to brace her tummy, suck it in hard, and then push back onto the hands and knees to lift off the pillow. Even though she did so, she shut her eyes tight and screwed her face up as she went.

Immediately after the treatment her forward bending was marginally improved. I expected little improvement at this stage since she was greatly visited by fear and the age-old belief that she should not bend. Her instructions for home were two lots of curl ups before bed that day (15 without stopping) and then again three times per day until I saw her again.

Second treatment

The second treatment was on day three. Frances was wary. Although she had been able to move better, her back was very sore with a different kind of raw and tender pain. She had also found it impossible to do the curl ups at home although her son had helped her. I immediately did some with her which she did well. For the time being, I suggested that she do them at home on her bed, which is always much easier.

Getting her into the prone position this time was not such a problem and I mobilised the stiff L5 segment for longer with pure forward and backwards gliding pressures from my hands. She became more comfortable and relaxed as I kept the pressure up. I then turned her over and did more curl ups which became more fluid and confident as she continued.

I repeated another short session of mobilising L5 but as it eased and felt more normal I switched to L4, the next level up. It was slightly stiff to lateral pressure directed to the right against the spinous process. I did this because I felt that this segment was involved to a lesser degree, and I knew that the muscle spasm would dissipate faster if more than one level was worked on.

L4 mobilisation was followed by another bout of curl ups, after which I lay her on a heat pad for ten minutes with her lower legs on a low stool.

Third treatment

The next treatment was a week later. I wanted Frances to get the tummy stronger with her own efforts at home and accordingly she had been bouncing the knees to the chest, rolling along the spine, and doing twenty curl ups every fours hours—morning, noon and night. I was thrilled to see her bowl through my front door, narrowly skirting around a table against the wall, like a ship in full sail. She had had much less pain although she was still not confident bending.

She had been industriously doing her mobilising and tummy strengthening at home and had progressed to doing the curl ups on the floor unaided, with her knees bent and feet wedged under a dresser.

The L5 segment felt so much looser and less guarded I decided to use my heel in her back to increase the force of the mobilisation. I put a pillow and paper sheet on the floor and asked Frances to lie over the pillow, quite close to the bed. Supporting myself with both hands on the bed I put my right foot across her buttocks.

The weight went through my foot and tilted the sacrum back, gapping the L5–S1 interspace. I maintained the pressure through my foot and rocked the pelvis gently from left to right. This was to relax the clench of the muscles so they would not contract suddenly to give her a sharp pain when more pressure was applied.

When the back was relaxed I slowly took all my weight on the right foot on the sacrum and placed my left heel on the spinous process of L5. With small oscillatory trampling movements I eased the age-old jamming between the bottom of the spine and the sacrum. Once she relaxed Frances found the pressure quite comfortable and could barely believe it was my full weight. I continued for only 60 seconds so there was minimal treatment soreness to discourage her next time.

> WARNING: Do not do this mobilisation at home.
> Allow only a qualified professional to undertake this treatment.

Frances was dispatched to continue her usual home routine. She had been shown how to squat which would continue the process of opening the back of the jammed L5–S1 spinal segment. This was to be repeated as many times a day as she could manage. I suggested she go for two short walks per day, squatting at various intervals along the way by holding onto a picket fence or anything which could take her weight.

Whenever she felt a twinge from her back she had to remember to stop what she was doing and squat This meant that she may have to do up to ten or twelve squats in a day, and I stressed that she could not overdo them (stiff grating knees subside in a day or so). She didn't have to do each squat for long, just a few seconds each time, pulling her tummy in, humping her low back and parting her knees wide so she could feel the sensation of her bottom dropping down off the base of her spine.

Fourth treatment

The next treatment was later that same week, in case there was any untoward reaction from the hefty mobilising. I repeated the treatment with the heel, doing a longer session during which she palpably relaxed more. I also used my heel transversely on L4 towards the right and it was a lot stiffer than I'd thought originally.

Frances was then introduced to the BackBlock routine to be continued at home on a daily basis—a particularly important development in her management. Its purpose was to reverse the underlying impaction of the base of the spine and correct her stooped kyphotic posture, both of which had led her to the state she was in.

Her lack of lumbar hollow meant that she was jarring the neurocentral core of her spine as she walked because it was unable to bow forward fleetingly to dissipate the impact of footfall. Her stoop was also creating strain on the base of the spine because the heavier upper part of her body was being carried too far in front of the base of her spine. Apart from helping restore a lordosis, we also needed the BackBlock to decompress the lower segments by pulling the pelvis longitudinally off the underside of L5.

I repeated the BackBlock three times with Frances, keeping to a maximum of 60 seconds. Any longer and her back would have become cast and it would have been too difficult (and painful) lifting her bottom off the Block. Frances was more supple than most and her legs draped back quite comfortably when she relaxed on the Block and her feet rolled outwards. However she did feel the habitual pulling sensation across the base of the spine which, like most people, she initially found unnerving.

Although the BackBlock is an integral part of all treatment regimens, I was very careful introducing it with Frances because her back was so close to being unstable at the bottom link. That being the case, we could not hurry. We had to strengthen her tummy beforehand, otherwise she would have had unusually severe pain getting off the Block each time. She also had to get started on her toe touching regimen, designed to strengthen the muscle power of the individual segments. This would happen next session.

I asked her to include the BackBlock in her exercise program at the end of each day, and I suggested she do it while watching the news on television, preferably after the children had gone to bed so she felt no need to hurry. I asked her to do three repetitions of 60 seconds on the BackBlock with bouncing her knees to her chest and fifteen curl ups each time afterwards. This takes about 15–20 minutes.

Fifth treatment

This treatment was several weeks later and Frances's back had been less painful, with lengthy periods painfree. However it still felt fragile, as if pain was never far away.

At this stage, it was important to embark on strengthening the intrinsic muscles of the spine to make her more secure bending. She had been improving her transversus abdominus with the curl ups (particularly the return journey to the floor by deliberate humping of the low back) and to be safe she needed an equal contribution from the deep spinal muscles as well.

I always introduce intrinsic strengthening late in the day because there is always reactive treatment soreness. (Patients should feel the benefit of their treatment before being put back into pain again.) I always start the strengthening with repeated toe touching exercises, except in cases of frank instability, where I do it as an unfurling action horizontally off the end of a table.

To do the toe touching from the standing position, I asked Frances to pull her tummy in hard (with a hand reinforcing it if necessary for security) and drop forward. At first she was loathe to go because her spine was so weak. To overcome this, I allowed her to climb down her legs with her hands until she could hang in the dropped forward position. Once there, she dangled her arms towards the floor and let her body relax for a few seconds.

To return upright she was instructed to pull her tummy in hard and tighten her buttocks to unfurl her spine to vertical, with her head coming up last. I asked her to repeat the exercise up to 15 times, dropping a little more loosely to the floor each time. To help her overcome her ingrained fear, I explained the forward bending part of the exercise is helpful in pulling out the stiffness of the muscles, and the return journey to vertical is where most of the strengthening comes in.

At the end of the treatment I told Frances to expect some stiffness in her back and possibly down the back of her thighs over the next few days. She had not bent properly for years so she should expect some reaction. The spine itself would be sore too, in a fragile sort of way, and the best way to relieve that was rolling over it for several minutes followed by a few more curl ups. This could be repeated whenever necessary during the day.

I always assume that the soreness in the back is a reaction of the neurocentral interspaces (particularly L5–S1) to the direct compression of multifidus pulling the segments up and back, and slotting them snugly in place on top of one another as the spine straightens. This fleeting, active compression of the vertebrae together may stir up residual inflammation of the segment.

I advised Frances that her toe touching exercise had to be done every treatment session after squatting and before her BackBlock routine. The squatting prepares the spine for bending by making it more supple and the Block afterwards distracts the spine and helps dissipate the soreness.

Before discharging Frances I implemented one last exercise. She needed to use the BackBlock under the thoracic part of her spine to help get her shoulders back and re-establish better equilibrium of her torso over her sacrum. This would reduce the chronic postural strain of L5 tipped forward on the pelvis.

I instructed her to use the BackBlock on its flattest side, lengthwise down the spine with the upper edge level with the top of her shoulders. As usual, it took a bit of trial and error to get it in the right place, and then I asked her to take her arms over her head.

This was to help un-hunch her upper back by stretching the pectoral muscles at the front of her chest which were tight and keeping her tethered over in a stoop. She only needed to stay on the Block for a minute or so, punctuating that time by taking the arms up, interlacing the fingers and turning the palms away. When she was finished, I asked her to roll off to the side of the Block like a log, instead of lifting straight up and straining her neck.

Afterwards she felt freer, with her body looser in its skin when she got up. Invariably people remark that they feel taller and can breathe easier after using the BackBlock behind the chest. It always feels very releasing.

I suggested to Frances at her last session that ideally she should continue her self treatment on a daily basis, even in an abbreviated form. If ever she hurt her back again, she should immediately lie down on the floor and rock her knees to her chest and roll along the spine. As soon as she could she should quickly try to do several curl ups.

3 Facet joint arthropathy

Facet joint arthropathy is wear and tear of the facet joints. After segmental stiffness, I believe it is the most common cause of low back pain.

WHAT IS FACET JOINT ARTHROPATHY?

The term 'arthropathy' covers the wide range of this disorder, from fleeting joint sprain of the capsular ligaments, right through to frank arthritis of the joints.

Breakdown of the facets comes about in several ways: when the disc between two vertebrae flattens, causing the upper vertebra to ride down on the lower one and jam the back compartment (just like letting air out of a car tyre makes it run along on its rim); it also develops when the facets have to overdo their preventative role, either restraining forward bending, or preventing twist of the segments in the low back.

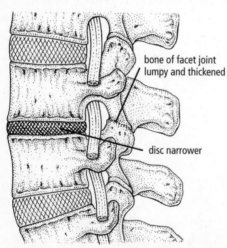

bone of facet joint lumpy and thickened

disc narrower

Figure 3.1 Facet arthropathy starts off as fleeting capsular strain, and ends up as frank joint destruction.

The lumbo-sacral facets are particularly taxed when the sacrum is permanently tipped forward, to cause a deep hollow in the low back (a lordosis or forward spinal curvature). Then the facets are forced to lock in apposition to stop the spine slipping forward off the sacrum. A leg length discrepancy can also affect several facets in the low back (and even into the thoracic spine and neck if the difference is great enough) as the lateral dip in the sacrum encourages the lumbar segments to slide sideways and twist.

However, attrition of the joints

caused by these background problems may take years to bring facet pain on. Trouble usually comes to the fore when lurking inflammation is provoked by additional small-scale injury. The slightest ricking or twisting incident, such as slipping on a shiny floor when you are turning to talk, or turning over in bed, can put a match to smouldering trouble and set it blazingly alight.

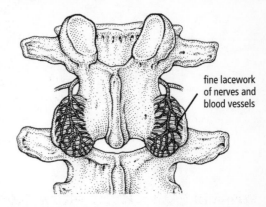

fine lacework of nerves and blood vessels

I believe capsular inflammation of the facets is very common and a potent source of backpain. Because the facet capsules play a heavy role in protecting the facets they are easily sprained. They act as tough elastic sleeves to absorb or dampen all jolts passing

Figure 3.2 Facet capsules are extremely bulky and are richly served with both blood and nerve supply.

through the facets, thus sparing them bone-to-bone bruising.

The facets are the most likely part of the spine to pull apart and come undone; in effect their sliding-apart freedom at the back of the spine is also their Achilles heel. The lumbar spinal segments have great difficulty controlling the first imperceptible degrees of bend-and-twist because there are so few diagonally criss-crossing ligaments and muscles to control the action (see Chapter 4). We depend on the disc being primed to give us this stability but the capsule too has to do what it can to fill the bill and be all things to all movements. The controlling of the joints and the sheltering them from impact means the facet capsules are constantly in the line of fire.

In most respects the capsules are admirably equipped to cope. They are incredibly elastic and strong with a rich blood supply to keep up running repairs. However the onerous protective role may cause one to bloat up angrily and compress the nearby spinal nerve. This causes a nasty sciatic pain down the leg.

The facet capsules have a prolific nerve supply to pick up any affront to the joint and relay it to the brain. However, the very sophistication of the nervous network may be part of the making of a back problem; the supersensitivity of the facet capsule may make it slightly too ready to invoke a reaction from its muscles.

This enthusiasm to protect the joint after it has suffered a strain can make a major problem out of a minor one. Thus a tiny wrench to your back when wrestling with a suitcase can lock you up for weeks when it should be gone in a day. On the other hand, supreme sensitivity from long-term joint pain may cause the muscles to reflexly underact, thus causing another set of problems.

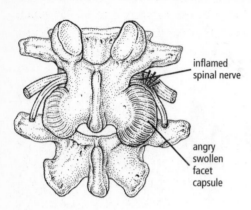

Figure 3.3 Capsular inflammation can readily irritate a nearby spinal nerve.

When the joint guarding is too attentive it jumps into action at the first sign of trouble. The nervous mechanism lights up and the muscles (presumably the local fibres of multifidus and the long superficial back muscles if the reaction is extreme) clench to protect it more. The prolonged muscle contraction can cause more inflammation, by slowing the flow of blood through the capsule. As the joint becomes more engorged it sends off more messages of pain to the brain and the protective cycle intensifies.

This over-reaction explains why it is so important to work through any minor discomfort and not allow it to get the better of you. It may also explain why the muscles stop acting altogether in cases of chronic facet pain. We know that multifidus in particular is underactive when the back has been painful for a long time and this may be another type of defence mechanism—this time deliberate underactivity to spare the super-sensitive joint added compression. Although the back may be more comfortable in the short term, in the long term there is a risk of introducing instability to the segment.

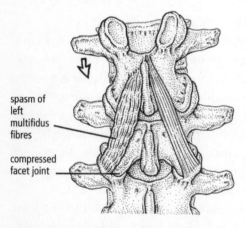

Figure 3.4 Sustained contraction (spasm) of multifidus can keep a facet joint engorged.

Whereas mild capsular strain is relatively easy to acquire, and fairly universal, true 'arthritic' change to the bony part of the facet is less common and may take years to become painful. Furthermore, I believe that even when arthritis is painful, its origins (certainly in the early stages) are 'capsular' rather than 'bone', at least until it gets to the point of actual bony destruction.

This may explain why treating advanced arthritic facets with the hands—in the way physiotherapists, osteopaths and chiropractors and some masseurs do—often relieves the pain. The accessing and handling of the tissues around a problem joint often interrupts the inflammatory cycle in a way which cannot be explained as doing things to the bone. Unlike the bone, capsular changes are more reversible and respond quite quickly to the comfort of suitable pressure.

Diagnosis by manual palpation

Just as with early stiffening of a spinal segment (Chapter 2), early capsular changes of the facets are only detectable via palpation with the hands, particularly the thumbs. Although the pain from an acutely inflamed joint may be crippling, routine imaging rarely shows anything. In the same way a twisted ankle is unlikely to show anything on a picture, the best way of telling if a facet is troublesome is by seeing whether it will move, by the way it feels, and by the way it responds to being handled.

Although not necessarily relevant in a self-help book such as this, it is interesting that human hands can tell such a lot about a facet problem. With early—otherwise undiagnosable—trouble with a facet the capsule feels like a dome of pulpy swelling under the skin when the thumbs probe in about 1.5 cm out to the side of the spine. If the problem is longstanding the capsule has a thickened leathery feel, caused by the chronic fibrosis, whereas a normal one will feel like nothing at all; health is conspicuous by its inconspicuousness. Experienced hands can also feel if there is overactivity of multifidus (it feels twangy, like an over-taut mini trampoline) or underactivity (when there is a leathery hollow where multifidus should be).

Once there are bony changes, palpation through the hands can tell how mobile (or immobile) the joint is and whether there is any crepitation, or grinding in the joint, as the joint surfaces move past one another. Again, this is not a finding which can be picked up any other way than manually, although in the neck you can often hear very loud chafing or rubbing from the joints as you turn your head. These palpatory findings are the preserve of professionals but they give a deeper understanding.

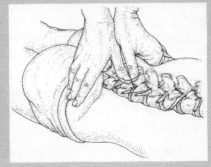

Figure 3.5 There is nothing better than human thumbs to feel the state of play of facet joints.

Once the joint surfaces become involved in the degenerative process, the changes stand out more clearly, even on X-rays. Because bone is radio-opaque, bony erosion can be seen, as can excess bone growth around the margins of the joint.

The pain is different in the different phases of the condition. Capsular pain is angry and mercurial, sometimes passing down the leg with different changes in position. By the time it has progressed to bony breakdown it is a deep-seated, gnawing ache which goes through like a meat cleaver in the side of your back, or across to the other side too if both joints of the segment are affected.

To confuse the issue, there may be no pain when the X-rays look absolutely awful. This is because there has *never* been a clear correlation between X-rays and degrees of pain. Sometimes the imaging films show nothing at all and yet a patient is genuinely crippled by pain. Somebody else's X-rays can look like a snow storm, with white roughed bone surfaces and strange knobbled outgrowths around margins of the joints, yet there has never been a day of pain. Hence the maxim of our practice: treat the patient not the X-rays.

CAUSES OF FACET ARTHROPATHY

1 Disc degeneration
- Disc stiffening allows the facet capsules to tighten
- Disc narrowing causes the facet joint surfaces to override

2 Abnormal posture
- A sway back causes the lower facets to jam
- Weak tummy muscles can jam the facets
- A shorter leg can cause arthritis of the facets

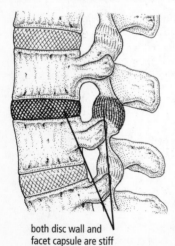

both disc wall and
facet capsule are stiff

Disc stiffening allows the facet capsules to tighten

The earliest form of stiffness of a facet joint may be nothing more than a fleeting protective spasm of its overlying multifidus muscle. A fluke odd movement, or an awkward posture for a while, and the muscle locks the joint temporarily to protect it. It is noticeable as a sore tight patch beside your spine which feels like a crimped link but which passes off within a day or two.

Figure 3.6 The facet capsules at the back of a segment can stiffen, alongside the disc at the front.

Even fleeting stiffness of the neurocentral core at the front of the segment can translate across to the strong capsular ligaments at the back. Because of the strength and toughness of their fibres, these ligaments are the first to lose stretch as the mobility of the front compartment declines. Even before obvious loss of disc height, disc immobility can greatly reduce the freedom of the facets.

In their less yielding state the capsular structures are much more vulnerable to injury. Their yanking with everyday movement amounts to repeated micro-trauma so that more and more capsular fibres are torn. On a microscopic scale there is oozing of blood and lymph into the interstitial spaces (between the fibres) where it lies about and gradually solidifies. This is scar tissue or adhesions. As the capsule becomes increasingly cobbled by adhesions it stiffens and the facet joint underneath loses play.

This augments the chain reaction fuelled by the facet joint as well. From now on, the back and front compartments of the segment contribute to the poor freedom of the upper vertebra articulating on the lower one. The stiffness of the link can be felt from the outside. It is less yielding to pressure as you roll back and forth over it and often feels like a plug of cement in a rubber hose. (Sometimes you can feel the stiffer facet by tipping from side to side.)

Disc narrowing causes the facet joint surfaces to override

As the disc becomes tighter it loses fluid and shrinks. As the disc narrows and the top vertebra rides down more on the lower one, the two facet surfaces come together in a tight uncomfortable fit. The top one can creep so far down the lower one that it digs into the neck of bone at the base and starts bearing weight.

From this point the joint's breakdown continues apace. The lining membrane of the capsule secretes greater amounts of synovial fluid to keep up the embattled lubrication and sluice the joint interfaces clean. The synovial fluid also carries large phagocytic cells which surround and devour each tiny particle of cartilage, and in this way the joint is kept in optimal running order. The greater the

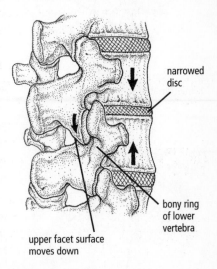

narrowed disc

bony ring of lower vertebra

upper facet surface moves down

Figure 3.7 The facet surfaces override when the disc space narrows.

internal friction of a joint the more synovial fluid is pumped in, like tears flooding the eyes to get rid of grit, until eventually the excess fluid becomes a problem in itself.

The fluid build-up can cause pain, but the tension of the joint may also invoke reflex contraction (spasm) of the multifidus muscle which lies immediately over top. As the muscle fibres shorten, the joint is held more firmly and compressed, increasing the pressure from the trapped fluid inside. Although this protective response has not been documented, I suspect it may account for the rapid alteration in the feel of a tense facet when it is touched by probing thumbs. The typical dome of capsular swelling can subside so quickly it feels as if a release valve has let the fluid escape. This may be multifidus letting go, allowing the joint to move freely, thus evacuating its fluid. I am always surprised by how quickly mobilising can bring this about and get rid of the pain.

A sway back causes the lower facets to jam

If the angle of the sacrum tips forward more than its average 50 degrees the spine is forced to hollow more as it arches back to the upright again. This causes inordinate wear of the lumbo-sacral facets. In some people the sacral angle can approach almost 90 degrees (with the sacral surface nearly vertical),

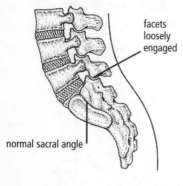

facets loosely engaged

normal sacral angle

and to keep the spine hooked on to the sacrum the two opposing surfaces of the L5–S1 facets remain permanently jammed. In effect the whole spine hangs on to the pelvis at these two bony hooks, like sash window catches, and this takes its toll.

The facet joints are not designed for this sort of heavy duty wear. The closedness of the joint surfaces is bad enough but their excessive grinding is much more destructive. With a normal lordosis the facets are in similar contact only when the spine is fully bent forward, although the posterior ligamentous lock, which comes into force when the back is fully rounded, shares some

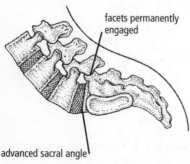

facets permanently engaged

advanced sacral angle

Figure 3.8 When the sacral angle is small, the lumbo-sacral facets are loosely engaged, but when the angle is steep they remain locked to keep the spine from slipping off the sacrum.

of the load. When an overly lordotic spine bends forward, the ligamentous lock cannot operate because the lumbar hollowing puts it on the slack (stressing again why it is so important to bend and lift with the back humped).

Excessive use of the facet stop-ramp puts the facets under all-day duress and abrades a continuous spume of cartilage off the joint surfaces. This gritty debris floats around in the joint space, acting as a micro-abrasive which scours down the residual cartilage surfaces even faster.

In extreme cases of lordosis, the upper facet surfaces override so far down the lower ones that the tips of the upper bony pillars come to rest at the base of the lower ones. The two fine prongs of bone projecting down from the vertebra above (the front of which provides the articulating surface) are no match for a disc when it comes to spreading load, and breakdown escalates.

Along with the bony changes, there can be marked soft tissue contracture of the joint capsules, in effect creating a bow-string which keeps the spine over-arched. As the fibres shorten and the roominess decreases, the joint surfaces become so close-packed they find it hard to pull away from each other to let the spine hump forward. This greatly reduces the bending freedom of the spine.

The backward arching action of the spine can become even more limited as the upper bony tips dig into the base, even jacking the interbody joint open as the spine tries to arch. If there is simultaneous impact of the foot hitting the ground as the back arches, the bony ring below can break. We see this as stress fractures of the spine with fast bowlers in cricket.

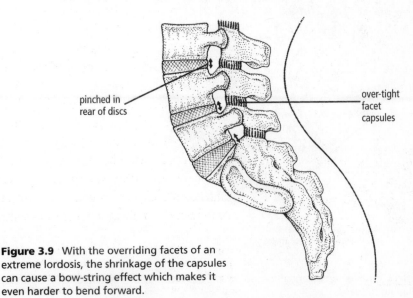

pinched in
rear of discs

over-tight
facet
capsules

Figure 3.9 With the overriding facets of an extreme lordosis, the shrinkage of the capsules can cause a bow-string effect which makes it even harder to bend forward.

In the long term, when the sacral angle remains marked, there is adaptive remoulding of the bone of the lower facet surface to create a bony impediment to the spine slipping forward. Similar to the way an unstable joint sprouts more bone around its edges to keep the facet in joint (see Chapter 6). Nature comes up with an ingenious way of making these joints more secure. A bar of bone forms across the lower facets to bolster their stop-ramp function, like bolting a steel bar across railway tracks. This minimises forward trespass of the spine on the sacrum.

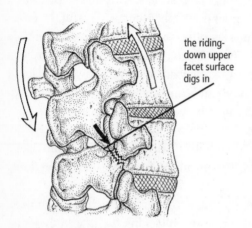

the riding-down upper facet surface digs in

Figure 3.10 Heavy impact while the back is arched can cause a fracture of the bony ring.

Strangely enough, the occupations which cause most facet trouble put the back into the fully stooped posture rather than an over-arched one. Shearers and farriers often spend hours bent double, with their facets fully engaged at the top of the stop-ramp. Initially this causes a ligamentous strain by stretching the fibrous capsules of the facets. Later on it causes bony degeneration from the grinding of the facet surfaces perpetually locked up against one another to keep the spine hooked on.

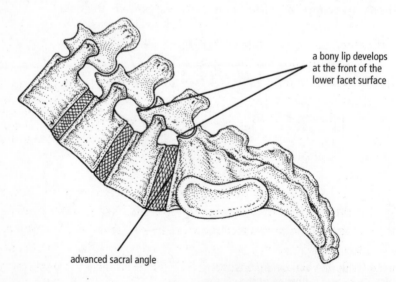

a bony lip develops at the front of the lower facet surface

advanced sacral angle

Figure 3.11 With extreme lumbar lordosis, the lower facet surfaces remould to prevent the spine slipping forward.

Weak tummy muscles can jam the facets

Weakness of the tummy can bring about a similar lordotic effect—but at least it is more under your control. As the tummy muscles weaken they often passively lengthen at the same time. As they stretch, they allow the front of the pelvis to tip down, causing a pronounced hollow in the low back. This causes the lumbo-sacral facets to engage, spending most of their time working as stop-ramps to prevent the rest of the spine sliding forward down the sacrum.

This is part of the explanation for backache which goes with pregnancy and ordinary old fat-tummy obesity. As the tummy gets bigger and more weight is carried in front of the line of gravity, the lower back goes into an even deeper hollow as you over-arch backwards to balance the weight out front. As the sacrum tips down, the lower lumbar facets lock into apposition to keep the spine on the pelvis. Abdominal strengthening to control the lordosis is an important part of the treatment of this problem.

A shorter leg can cause arthritis of the facets

Most of us have one leg shorter by a millimetre or two, which I believe is a common cause of backpain. A shorter leg places great strain on the low facets to hold the spine locked in place on the pelvis. The greater the discrepancy, the greater the diagonal sideways-and-forwards trespass of the spine down the sacrum.

The spine slips forward as well as sideways because the hip joint lies in front of the centre of gravity. Thus on the side of the shorter leg the pelvis dips down at the front as well as laterally on that side. The combination of the two aberrant tendencies causes great wear and tear on all lumbar facets but the lumbo-sacral ones in particular.

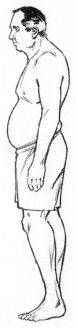

Figure 3.12 A lax abdominal wall lets the front of the pelvis down so the low back over-arches.

The mechanics of distortion are more complicated than first imagined because the vertebrae then rotate around a central axis of movement, as well as slipping diagonally across the sacrum. A new centre of movement comes into effect as the facet on the downhill side engages and the vertebra swings around this new pivot to twist further. All this makes for complicated movement of the bottom vertebra when one leg is shorter.

Furthermore, the hip joint of the longer leg develops trouble too. It acquires a tightness at the front of the joint because that leg always stands with the knee bent. This drops down that side of the pelvis and equalises the sit of the sacrum. The hip tightness makes the stride of both legs uneven. Because it cannot angle backwards, the spine has to compensate while walking by twisting more to that side to even up the steps. With all of us taking thousands of steps per day, you can see the spine must repeatedly twist one way as we walk. All in all, the spine has a rich cocktail of irritations where it joins the sacrum.

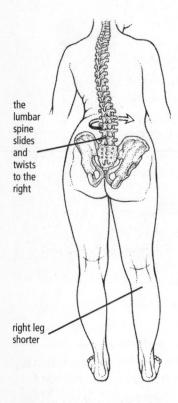

the lumbar spine slides and twists to the right

right leg shorter

Figure 3.13 With a shorter right leg, the spine creeps diagonally forward and sideways down the sacrum. When the downhill (R) facet engages, the spine pivots around it as it twists to the right.

It is not really possible to be pedantic about which facet will be the most painful at the lumbo-sacral level, although there is a rule of thumb that the facet on the side of the shorter leg will be painful in the early years while the side of the longer leg will be more painful later in life.

With extreme discrepancies, the downhill facet ingeniously remoulds in a similar fashion to the remoulding in an over-lordotic spine. In what are termed 'wrap-around bumpers', the lower facet surface develops bony outgrowths to stabilise the lateral trespass of the upper vertebra. Although these excess knobbles of bone can look frightening on X-rays, they are no indication of pain.

This 'facet tropism' or asymmetry of the lumbar facets is an issue which causes great excitement in academic circles. However, I believe the high incidence of differing leg lengths explains the prevalence of tropism. It is the readiness of the spine to adapt to the anomalous sit of the sacrum (especially if there is too much lordosis as well) which accounts for the dissimilarity between two paired joints.

Tropism has been unearthed by researchers who have been quick to point out its strong link to backpain. As a shop floor clinician, I see things from the other perspective: the facets *become* different to help reduce backpain when the legs are born unequal in length, rather than the facets themselves *being* different at birth and causing backpain. This should banish your despair on being told you have backpain because your lumbar facets are dissimilar. I see leg length inequality as a highly significant factor in the genesis of backpain—although conventional wisdom decrees that differences of less than 2 cm are unimportant—a verdict I deplore.

Correcting leg length discrepancies by using a heel raise in the shoe of the shorter leg is an early and mandatory part of self treatment. Only an approximate adjustment is necessary; it is better not to jack up the difference to the nearest millimetre. Since you have coped for so long with one leg shorter, the difference should be minimised rather than fully corrected—or it simply adds another set of strains to the pre-existing ones.

Golf clinic

As a result of the rotation involved, golf can often traumatise the facets joints because of their role in limiting spinal twist. As a right-handed golfer swings to the left, the row of facets down the right side of the spine jam up against each other like doors against a door jam. The facets down the left side of the spine pull apart. The forcible closing on one side and wrenching open on the other can cause breakdown.

Serious golfers will cause less damage, and get a better swing, if they take the twist higher in their back. From waist level up, the facet alignment is different and no longer stops the vertebrae swivelling. If golfers employ the 'flying elbows' technique of taking the twist in an arching spiral up the back, they will not only avoid damaging the facets but hit a better shot.

THE WAY THIS BACK BEHAVES

The acute phase

The high-pitched crisis of acute facet inflammation usually follows a wrenching of the spine which provokes a slower brewing problem. A dormant stiff facet sets itself up for being hurt by not accepting shock as readily as its neighbours above and below—or even its facet partner on the other side.

The cause of the flare up can be hard to pinpoint but in a matter of hours the injury can be literally crippling. It is usually something awkward but not disastrous, such as lifting a pot plant which was heavier than you thought. You often hear a small sound, like a click or a small tear in your back, which may give you fleeting pain at the time but then passes off. But by nightfall or next morning when the heat of the exertion has gone a nasty frightening back pain comes on.

At the height of the crisis, the symptoms are a stabbing pain in the side of the back which often goes with searing waves of pain down your leg. Your back feels hard and sore with muscle spasm on one side but the leg pain can be almost unbearable. The pain is often associated with intense pins and needles and a burning sensation which floods downwards as your leg takes weight.

Leg pain of this type is called sciatica, but it is different from the sciatica of a bulging disc (see Chapter 5). Although it is hard for you to know the difference, as a rule, acute facet inflammation gives a hot surging tide of prickling pain down the leg, whereas disc prolapse sciatica is more like intense cramp locking up the leg muscles.

Manual diagnosis of an acutely inflamed facet

Locating the swollen joint with the thumbs usually confirms the facet as the source of trouble. Probing in beside the spine with the thumbs, the inflamed capsule can be felt welling up from below, like the dome of a cathedral rising out of low-lying cloud. It has the typically tense feel of an over-filled hot water bottle, and will rebuff the pressure of the thumbs.

Apart from the joint feeling hard under the skin, direct pressure usually gives a sudden slice of pain through the back which may then flood down the leg. Unlike this direct evidence of facet involvement, it is impossible to be so sure if the disc is causing sciatica. The disc is around at the front of the spine, out of reach of the hands and, I feel, can only be assumed to be the culprit if there is nothing wrong with the facets. I mention this because there was a time, not too long ago, when all forms of sciatica were deemed to come from herniated or bulging discs. I believe discogenic sciatica is infinitely rarer than facet-based sciatica—though much harder to fix.

Typical facet joint sciatica is easily set off by changes in position. Any posture which compresses the swollen joint can exacerbate the pain. Even small positional adjustments can cause a corresponding reaction down the leg, as if the new contortion increases the swelling on the nerve. The pain then fades as the swelling oozes to other parts of the joint capsule and drains away.

In the acute stage of facet arthropathy there is usually armour-plated spasm of the muscles protecting the back. Unfortunately the spasm often makes matters worse by obliterating too much movement and letting the swelling accumulate. Often the best course of action is to take anti-inflammatory drugs to reduce the heat, and then muscle relaxants to break the cycle of muscle holding.

This treatment is especially indicated if your spine is listing over, with the hips protruding one side and shoulders the other. This 'windswept' deformity is known as sciatic scoliosis and is caused by the muscles on one side of the spine contracting more than the other. Even though its purpose is to spare the joint, the resulting discord often makes the spine more susceptible to other injury, and makes the current problem harder to fix. At this stage, the best thing to do is take your medication and do gentle knee-rocking exercises in bed to 'milk' the joint.

With severe facet inflammation, the recovery from the acute stage is usually quite rapid—as long as the muscle spasm does not hang on for too long. Fear at this stage is usually the greatest cur and can slow recovery significantly, sometimes completely. Excessive agitation or anger (even if it is subconscious) will also lower the pain threshold and create a 'volitional' tension in the muscles on top of the automatic protective one.

All going well, the back is not excessively plagued by anxieties and the muscle spasm releases the joint to get going. As soon as normal movement returns, the joint will be well on the way to recovery; and the sooner the better. Normal movement 'works' the joint properly and disperses the inflammation, and everything assumes normality again. Normality begets normality.

What causes the acute pain?

The facet's response to injury is the same as any other of the body's synovial joints. When a knee or ankle is twisted there is a sudden jerk of pain the moment you do it, and just after it feels wonky but still workable. Within a few hours it becomes more painful as the joint swells. It may reach a peak after a period of inactivity when you suddenly sense the pain stubbornly roosting there and you cannot work it away.

An injured facet joint behaves in exactly the same way. But because of the closer quarters inside the back, with many moving parts of spinal machinery packed cheek by jowl into a tightly confined space, a minor injury can have devastating effects. With so many sensitive structures (not least the spinal nerve) and so little room for anything to swell, a relatively small mishap can cause a crisis.

When a facet joint is wrenched, the synovial lining of the capsule weeps clear fluid into the joint space. It is similar to the way tears well up in the eyes, except the tension of the fluid trapped inside the joint is much more problematic. The engorgement makes the joint semi-rigid from its own bloatedness and it has difficulty sliding and gapping open. The lack of movement makes it less competent at pumping out the fluid, which consequently accumulates even faster. Eventually pressure from the swelling in the joint causes pain.

As with all joints, special 'mechano-receptors' in the capsular wall are stimulated by the pressure of the fluid, and messages relayed to the brain are interpreted as pain. Pain is also registered by the leakage of inflammatory fluids from the torn tissue of the original joint injury. As their chemical concentration rises, free nerve endings in the joint capsule are stimulated. These are called 'chemo-receptors' and they send off more messages to the brain about pain.

The typical searing pain down the leg is caused by irritation of the nerve root when it becomes embroiled in the joint's inflammation, simply by being so close. As it makes its way past the joint on its way out of the spine it is both physically squashed by the swollen capsule and chemically irritated by the cocktail of toxins coming from its inflamed wall. Things hot up apace when the nerve starts to chafe where it threads past both the capsule and other swollen structures. Eventually it too becomes inflamed and leaks inflammatory fluid.

Interrupting the pain cycle

When I palpate an acute spine I cannot feel much at all because the superficial muscle spasm is too unyielding to allow the hands to penetrate. Before proceeding, I induce muscle relaxation by getting the patient to rock the knees to the chest and then rolling back and forth over the facet. (Curl up exercises do it faster if they are not too uncomfortable to do). The physical movement 'pumps' the joint clear by providing artificial activity to evacuate the fluid. This lowers the tension in the tissues and interrupts the cycle of pain. In the same way that a twisted ankle becomes more comfortable when the swelling subsides and movement resumes, the pain of an acute facet problem dramatically reduces as the engorged joint empties.

The pain also fades as fresh blood passes through the joint, cleansing away toxins liberated by the damaged tissues. As the stale blood is dispersed it lowers the concentration of metabolites and reduces the potency of the pain messages to the brain.

The chronic phase

Chronic inflammation of a facet joint causes a local patch of pain beside the spine. It typically welcomes the piercing pressure from your own fist or fingers on the spot. Although the joint is several centimetres below the skin it can be felt quite easily, like a brick under a mattress, and you can often elicit a half relieving sweet pain through your own digging. It usually feels about the size of a squash ball.

Lessening the pain

Depending on the nature of the inflammation, a facet problem may be relieved by stretching or compressing the joint. If there is established tightness and inelasticity of the capsule, you may get relief by leaning away from the pain and pulling the joint apart. Although the stretching discomfort hurts at the time, the back feels freer and looser afterwards, with less pain. If the problem is more acute, with trapped engorgement in the facet capsule, it can be eased by leaning towards the pain and closing the joint down. This gives a sharper, more piercing pain which can be almost unbearable for a moment but again feels better afterwards. If you arch backwards while still leaning over to the painful side, you can create an even shriller pain, like a knife going in. Alarming as it sounds, compressing the joint like this helps evacuate it and takes some of its bursting discomfort away.

You will see in the self-help section that milking an engorged joint is an integral part of treatment. You can use a Ma Roller on the floor to do this (the purchasing details for which are at the back of the book). By lying on your back on the floor and rolling back and forth over the roller with the knees bent, you get the familiar sweet pain as the pressure empties the joint. Take care not to inflame the facet. The Ma Roller is tough medicine when a facet is very irritable and it is easy to stir things up. Do not remain on it more than a few seconds.

It is safer to use a tennis ball when the condition is very inflamed, because it is safer and kinder on the joint. Its pressure is the nearest thing to the direct contact from human thumbs. But remember it too can make the joint sore and should never be continued for longer than 60 seconds, three times per week.

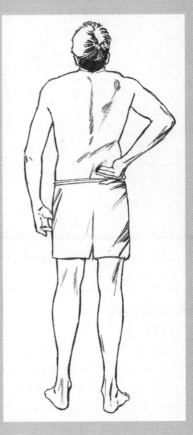

Figure 3.14 Facet problems seem to yearn for the piercing pressure of hands.

What causes the chronic pain?

Most of the pain from a chronically inflamed facet joint comes from the stretching of the stiff soft tissues around the joint. As a sequel to disc thinning and overriding of facet surfaces, there is adaptive shortening of the capsule and the soft issues which reinforce it.

'Mechano-receptors' situated in the capsule wall detect the tension in the soft tissues as they are pulled. As small spherical structures between the tissue fibres, they are squashed like tiny ping-pong balls under guitar strings as the tension in the capsular wall mounts. The messages are again relayed to the brain and interpreted as pain.

As an isolated joint becomes tighter and more crimped in the chain it becomes chronically painful. Its capsule is less able to pay out and stretch with the other links in the spine as your body bends and sways about. At a certain point the tightness becomes so unforgiving that every movement elicits a response from the pain receptors embedded in the over-tight fibres.

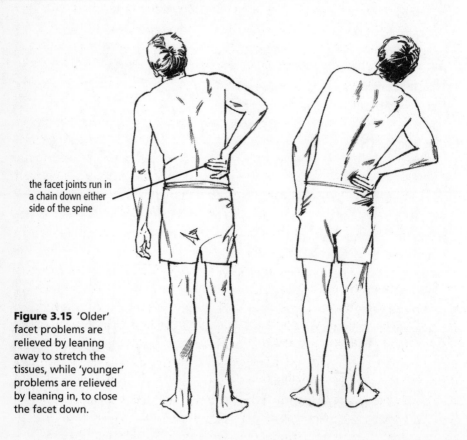

the facet joints run in a chain down either side of the spine

Figure 3.15 'Older' facet problems are relieved by leaning away to stretch the tissues, while 'younger' problems are relieved by leaning in, to close the facet down.

At this stage, the crimped link is extremely susceptible to additional injury. Its lack of stretch causes fibres of the tight capsule to be tweaked by any chance movement passing through the spine. As each shock racks through, all the mobile segments ride out the force, like a row of corks dancing on the water as a wave passes underneath, except the stiff one which is wrenched anew. This adds insult to injury. Chemo-receptors in the joint capsule are activated by substances released from the torn tissue fibres and their constant bathing of the free nerve endings means the joint emits a barrage of pain signals.

With micro-trauma heaped upon a pre-existing stiffness the familiar old pain becomes a different sort of pain. There is a low grade tenderness in your back and a newer pain in the leg. Pain in the buttock and thigh comes and goes with activities which increase the pressure on the facets, such as slumped sitting or prolonged bending activities like gardening. This is called referred pain. The mechanism for this pain is not the same as the direct inflammation of the nerve root which we saw in the acute disorder. Referred pain is a complex phenomenon where structures sharing the same nerve supply as the inflamed joint 'mistakenly' feel pain too. In the same way that the pain of a heart attack is felt in the neck and left arm, nowhere near the heart, the referred pain from an irritable facet joint can be felt quite far away from the point of trouble.

Referred pain rarely extends below the knee although other symptoms can. These can be diffuse, sometimes indefinable sensations which are difficult to put a name to. One leg may not work as well as the other; it is the typical 'gammy' leg and may feel heavier as you walk. The back of the thigh may feel sensitive when you sit, as if the skin and subcutaneous fat is thinner. One foot may feel colder, or as if you have a pebble in your shoe. Sometimes the heel feels numb, or ants seem to be crawling up your calf. Sometimes it feels as if a cobweb is brushing your skin or the leg hairs prickle uncomfortably against your trousers. The buttock of your bad side may feel bonier when you sit, or the hamstring muscle of the problem side tighter. When you bend forward, there may be a tension beside the spine, down through the buttock and into your leg which makes the knee bend automatically as you go over.

Almost all of these signs vary from day to day, sometimes from hour to hour, and almost from one position to the next. They can be explained as the effect of variable swelling within the facet joint capsule. Another explanation points to the build-up of pressure around the nerve root, impinging upon different sensory pathways in the nerve which brings about a wide variety of symptoms.

If there is protective muscle spasm guarding the stiff link, there will be some discomfort coming from the chronically stiffened muscles. This pain is typically a tired cramping feeling, made much worse by emotional 'tension'. Being 'uptight' increases the spinal symptoms by adding to the compression of the spine and congestion of the problem inside.

WHAT YOU CAN DO ABOUT IT
The aims of self treatment for facet joint arthropathy

With facet joint trouble, the primary objectives are to raise the height of the disc and relieve the congestion of the joint; and then make it run more smoothly. In the acute phase the joint is extremely irritable and treatment is designed to 'milk' it of its swelling. The technique of rocking the knees to the chest will do this. Once the joint is emptier and less painful, pivoting on the problem level helps mobilise it. The curl up exercises work it actively. Curl ups usually bring about a dramatic reduction in pain because the raised abdominal tone lifts the spine off the painful joint. Curl ups also relieve congestion by subjecting the joint to the normal contracting and relaxing of the muscles around it. Briefly using the tennis ball at this stage can also reduce the facet joint swelling, but care must be taken because it is easy to make things worse. You do this by lying on your back on the floor, knees bent, and positioning the ball under the sore spot. Roll back and forth on the ball, and press the pain away.

In the chronic phase the treatment is much more vigorous. It is aimed at stretching the inelastic joint capsule into its extremes of range. This promotes joint lubrication and cartilage repair by alternately closing down and pulling apart the joint. The rapid alterations in pressure contact of the joint surfaces also encourages a better 'circulation' through the cartilage bed. The Cobra– Pose of the Child exercise does this. Rolling on a tennis ball or Ma Roller pummels a tight joint capsule and gives the joint more freedom to move.

In the final stages of treatment, disimpaction of the neurocentral core is the ultimate objective. The BackBlock achieves this, and also restores an optimal lumbar hollow. It does this by stretching the front of the hips (the hip flexors) thus reducing an exaggerated lordosis, but it can also correct a pronounced lumbar kyphosis (less commonly a background factor with this condition) by stretching the anterior longitudinal ligament down the front of the spine. While on the Block it is often useful to rotate the pelvis in a minute twisting action which helps disengage the facets.

Ordinary toe touches are also important. These stretch shrunken facet capsules which, in the case of an exaggerated lordosis, exert a bow-string effect to keep the spine hollowed.

Ultimately, diagonal toe touches pull a tethered nerve root free of adhesions in the small exit-canal (or foramen) which may have developed from longstanding inflammation. These exercises also enhance the function of multifidus. The vigour of the action makes the muscles relax properly as the spine goes down and then works them on the way up. Their re-education helps restore joint perfusion (circulation of fluids) and leads to better control in the opening and closing of all lumbar facets.

A typical treatment for acute facet joint arthropathy

(See Chapter 7 for descriptions of all exercises and the correct way to do them.)

Purpose: Disperse joint swelling and inflammation, relieve muscle spasm

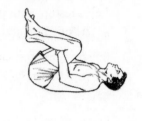

Rocking knees to the chest (60 seconds)

Rest (30 seconds)

_____

Rocking knees to the chest

Rest

_____

Rocking knees to the chest

Rest

_____

Rocking knees to the chest

Rest

_____

Reverse curl ups (five times)

Rest

_____

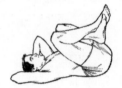

Reverse curl ups

Rest

_____

Reverse curl ups

Rest

_____

Rest in bed and use medication under the direction of your doctor. NSAIDS are particularly effective in reducing the pain from the inflamed joint so painkillers are not usually necessary. Repeat exercises every 2 hours throughout the day. When resting, you may be more comfortable in the foetal position with a pillow between the knees to decompress the joint.

For how long? You can progress to the sub-acute regimen when there is no flooding pins and needles pain down the leg, either when standing up from sitting or when taking weight on the leg. This can take a week to ten days, though it may be sooner.

A typical treatment for sub-acute facet joint arthropathy

Purpose: Disperse inflammation, relieve muscle spasm, disengage the jamming of the segments

Rocking knees to the chest (for 60 seconds)
Rolling along the spine (15–30 seconds)
Curl ups (five times)
Rest

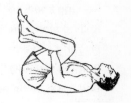

Rocking knees to the chest
Rolling along the spine (pivoting on sore spot)
Curl ups
Rest

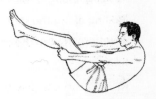

Rocking knees to the chest
Rolling along the spine
Curl ups
Rest

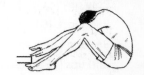

Rocking knees to the chest
Rolling along the spine
Curl ups
Rest

Repeat the regimen three times daily. After each session, rest on the floor for ten minutes with your lower legs supported on a sofa or soft chair, and a pillow under your head. Do not be alarmed if pivoting on the problem level causes a sharp pain in the back, or even leg pain. When up and about, avoid sitting in one position, or standing for too long. (This will usually bring on the pain down the leg.) Have two brief walks per day (less than fifteen minutes): you should walk tall and light and let your hips swing freely so the low back twists from left to right.

For how long? You should progress to the chronic treatment regimen when there is no leg pain. This usually takes a week to ten days but it may be much sooner.

A typical treatment for chronic facet joint arthropathy

Purpose: Decompress spine, mobilise facet joint, strengthen tummy, encourage cartilage regeneration

Rocking knees to the chest (60 seconds)

Rolling along the spine (15–30 seconds)

Pivoting on vertebra (15 seconds)

Rest (30 seconds)

Curl ups (five times)

Rocking knees to the chest

Rolling along the spine

Pivoting on vertebra

Rest

Curl ups

Cobra (10 seconds)

Pose of the Child (10 seconds)

BackBlock (60 seconds)

Rocking knees to the chest (30 seconds)

Curl ups (15 times)

Cobra

Pose of the child

BackBlock

Rocking knees to the chest

Curl ups

Tennis ball on sore joint (15 seconds)

Repeat program every day, morning or evening, and continue with NSAIDS (anti-inflammatories). At this stage you can often feel the soreness of the joint in the side of your back and the muscles clenching if it gets too congested. You can usually relieve the discomfort by rolling on your spine and pivoting on the painful joint at intervals through the day.

For how long? You may remain in this phase for several weeks as the joint slowly gets more mobile and less inclined to bloat up. You progress to the next regimen when your back simply feels 'dry' and tight down one side, with a stretching sensation in the buttock and leg when you bend forward.

A typical treatment for sub-chronic facet joint arthropathy

Purpose: Decompress spine, stretch the nerve root and adhesions, mobilise the joint to its extremes of range, strengthen the intrinsic spinal muscles (multifidus), encourage cartilage regeneration

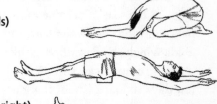

Cobra (for 10 seconds)
Pose of the child (for 10 seconds)
BackBlock (for 60 seconds)
Rocking knees to the chest (30 seconds)
Curl ups (15 times)

Cobra
Pose of the child
BackBlock (with pelvic swivel left and right)
Rocking knees to the chest
Curl ups

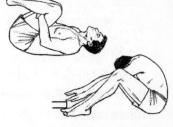

Cobra
Pose of the child
BackBlock (with pelvic swivel left and right)
Rocking knees to the chest
Curl ups

Floor Twists (two to bad side: one to good)
Ma Roller (15 seconds)

Diagonal toe touches (four times bad side: one good)
Squatting (30 seconds)

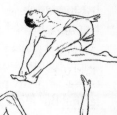

Diagonal toe touches
Squatting

Repeat program every day, morning or evening (tennis ball three times per week only). The pain and tightness in your buttock and the back of your thigh will often persist for a few days after the diagonal toe touching exercises. This is a natural reaction to stretching the nerve root free of its adhesions. If your leg gets too sore you may go back to the sub-acute regimen and resume taking the anti-inflammatories (NSAIDS) for a few days. This physical regimen continues indefinitely.

A CASE HISTORY OF FACET JOINT ARTHROPATHY

Sally is a 44-year-old Englishwoman who had complained of intermittent backache since she lifted a wheelbarrow while gardening eight years ago. The pain had been across her lower back, slightly more on the right side.

She is a woman of trim build who has her own freelance art advisory service. Over the years she had sought a multitude of treatments but eventually found the best way of keeping her pain under control was simply keeping fitter with aerobics classes and walking every day.

For two weeks prior to seeing me she had suffered increasing stiffness in her back. She related it to driving her car after one of her sons had altered the angle of the seat. It became more uncomfortable after an aerobics class and next morning she awoke with a new, severe pain on the outside of her right ankle which she described as 'like a headache of the ankle'.

She did not recall specifically hurting her back in the class but within a few days, after a 24-hour flight to Australia, the ache became like a 'drilling' sensation in the outside of her foot. It was relieved by activity and walking around, and made worse by sitting. Even small variations in the angle of a chair would increase or decrease the pain in her foot. Driving had become practically intolerable.

Her spinal movements were restricted, especially when she bent forward. I noted there was a flattening of the lumbar curve to the right of her low lumbar spine. She was nervous when asked to bend forward and had always tried to avoid doing this. Because of her general suppleness, I suspected that her limitation of movement was more from hesitation than spinal stiffness. Her back looked weak and trembled slightly as she went over.

When I palpated her spine she exhibited the typical central tubular stiffness of the neurocentral core, especially where the fifth lumbar vertebra joined the sacrum. My pressure was uncomfortable with the typical 'bruised bone' feeling but it did not reproduce her familiar foot pain.

On the other hand, the facet joint of L5–S1 on the right had a tense engorged feel with a piercing knife-like pain as I probed down through its swollen capsule. However, my pressure on the facet (out to the side and slightly lower than the spinous process of L5) did not reproduce her ankle pain, which I might have expected. Neither did testing the tension on her sciatic nerve by raising her straight leg off the bed to beyond 90 degrees.

MRI scans of Sally's back revealed a much diminished disc space between L5 and the sacrum, and a moderate bulging of the disc wall. Her X-rays also showed early degenerative (arthritic) change of both lumbo-sacral facets. Her provisional diagnosis had been 'acute disc prolapse'.

My conclusions were that the bruised sensitivity of L5 had probably always been there and was indicative of an impacted L5. I also felt that the moderate disc bulge of L5 was not the cause of her ankle pain, and she did not have an 'acute disc'. I deduced this because her sciatic nerve was not sensitive to the straight leg raise (SLR) testing, indicating that the nerve itself was not inflamed. I surmised the disc was bulging simply because it was being compressed by the muscle spasm protecting the painful segment. A perfect case of the disc doing as it should: acting as a shock absorber. Since only the facet joint with its superior nerve supply (and not the disc which has very little) is capable of referring pain far into the leg, it was much more likely that her pain came from her facet joint, not the disc.

I felt that Sally's ankle pain was the result of inflammation of the right facet after it had taken the brunt of some recent minor twisting trauma at her aerobics class. This had immediately followed her back being stirred up by the altered angle of her driving seat. I also assumed the much reduced disc space at L5–S1 had predisposed her to injury of the facets through the long-term overriding of the joint surfaces.

First treatment

I gently mobilised the tense and swollen facet with my thumbs and it evacuated rapidly in the typical way, like letting water out of an over-filled hot water bottle. Within moments the capsule had lost its tension and developed the nothingness of a normal joint.

Joint mobilisation was followed by several minutes of gently rocking Sally's knees to her chest with the ankles crossed, all the time attempting to gap open the back of the spine. This was done to help further disperse the swelling in the joint but also to stretch out protective muscle spasm of both the superficial and deep muscles of the spine.

Assisted curl ups were then started with Sally's knees bent and me sitting on her feet helping her up. Sally was anxious because of the pain (which is commonly the case) and had great difficulty getting up the first time. Tucking her chin in and rounding her lower back made it more comfortable. After the first two or three they became easier. However the quality and the smoothness of the curl ups continued to improve after each successive session of rocking her knees. In the first treatment Sally did approximately ten curl ups each time over a twenty minute period with rests in between. After each rest she resumed bouncing her knees to her chest for a couple of minutes before doing more curl ups.

The benefits from the curl ups are diverse. On a basic level, the action of rolling up along the spine helps to mobilise the block of lumbar segments which have been stiffened by the protective hold of the muscles. At a more high-tech level, the strenuous activity of the abdominal muscles helps switch off the over-activity of the back muscles and so lessens the muscle spasm in the back. A third benefit of the strong tummy work is raising the intra-abdominal pressure which elongates the spine from within and helps offset the impaction of its base.

Sally went home with instructions to take an increased dose of anti-inflammatories. These tablets are very effective in treating the pain of facet arthropathy but less so with discogenic pain. She was also to repeat the knees rocking and curl ups twice more that day before going to bed and then repeat them the next day at four hourly intervals. Each knee bouncing and curl ups regimen was to last approximately twenty minutes.

Sally felt freer in the back the day after the first treatment and the ankle pain was not as gnawing. She also had a more comfortable early evening but was very stiff and in pain again on waking the next day. Although she attempted to dissipate the pain by rocking her knees and doing the curl ups as instructed, she was unable to get relief.

I assumed that the increase in her pain had come about through the gradual refilling of the joint overnight so that it was swollen and tense again by morning. Perhaps some resumption of the protective muscle spasm of multifidus may have played a part in this, but it is impossible to say whether this caused the joint bloating.

Second treatment

I did not see Sally again until day three although it would have been better to do so the very next day.

Her forward bending was not improved from day one but the joint was less tense when it was palpated and there was less of a 'held' feel around the L5 segment. This meant that I could feel more clearly through to the neurocentral junction of L5–S1.

I briefly mobilised L5 centrally by repetitively gliding it forward on the sacrum with my thumbs and releasing it. It gave the typical sweet pain under pressure but did not reproduce the pain in the right ankle. I did this before mobilising the injured facet because I knew that the facet would move apart more freely if I released the central core of the joint first.

When I felt her right facet joint it was less swollen. This meant the joint's function was less obscured by the recent swelling and I could feel down more to the chronic limitation of its mobility, which had probably been there for years. When I did this the nature of the pain changed: it was not so piercing and, although still uncomfortable, it had a more agreeable quality. (I am never concerned when patients report this sort of pain because I know it releases endorphines, the body's natural opiates, and although it hurts at the time it feels better afterwards.)

The rest of the treatment consisted of knee rocking and more curl ups, to a total of approximately thirty, and when she left I asked her to continue these at home.

Third treatment

Over the intervening four days the pain had been up and down, with some painfree periods. It was still easy to set the pain off by sitting awkwardly or getting tired. Sally was moving more freely and no longer walked in a slightly waddling fashion with her bottom out. She was better able to gain relief by rocking her knees to her chest and doing curl ups—always a memorable milestone.

On palpation the facet had completely lost its tense swelling and had reverted to the typical leathery feel of the joint capsule. (It had probably felt like that for years.) Her forward bending movement was more flowing and the flattened patch over the right lumbo-sacral area had gone.

Most of the treatment could now be directed to the central jamming of L5, which I used my heel to mobilise. Sally lay on the floor over a pillow with her hands under her tummy. Leaning on the bed with both hands, I placed my right foot across her buttocks, below the coccyx, to take my weight and the left heel on the spinous process of L5. By transferring weight with small oscillatory trampling movements between both feet, the segment was gently worked free.

> WARNING: Do not do this mobilisation at home.
> Allow only a qualified professional to undertake this treatment.

The purpose of deeper mobilisation pressures is to loosen the jammed L5 segment at the base of the spine. The added force of using my foot glides the vertebra forward, with much less discomfort because the pressure (although far greater than using the hands) is distributed over a wider area. Each trample pulls up and releases the stiffened fibrous rim of the L5 intervertebral disc, which sucks fluid in and restores pliability to the neurocentral core.

As L5 started to release centrally I then used my heel on the right facet which is harder to feel with the foot. Rather, it is sensed as thickening or sludge in the gully between the ledge of pelvic bone and the spinous process. At no time did central pressure or the facet pressure reproduce Sally's ankle pain (which it often does). After the treatment she felt lighter in the body and walked freer, swinging her hips.

Sally went home with instructions on how to do her own form of central core mobilising of L5 by rolling back and forth along the spine.

I asked her to include several minutes of spinal rolling before she did her knee rocking exercise and the curl ups. The slightly longer routine was to be repeated twice throughout the day but more frequently if her back started to stiffen.

Fourth treatment

The next treatment was ten days later and Sally reported longer painfree periods. The pain was less severe and disappeared more rapidly. More importantly, she was able to rid herself of pain when it returned.

To provide her with the ultimate means of rehydrating the lumbo-sacral disc, I instructed her in the use of a BackBlock. On the first treatment she could not tolerate it well at all, even on its flattest side. When it was under her sacrum she found it difficult to relax and let both legs drop down to the floor so her spine pulled out. She found the pulling sensation across her low back unnerving, and after only a few seconds she wanted to put one foot on the floor and bend her knee. This was a sufficient sign to remove the Block, bring both knees to the chest, rocking them gently to ease the spine, and then, once her back was looser, go on to do ten curl ups. The tri-partite routine was repeated twice, so in the end she had done 30 curl ups.

I explained to Sally that this routine would now become part of her life. Ideally it was to be repeated at the end of each day but more so if her back was getting cast and sore during the day. If her leg pain returned, she should not try to get rid of it by using the Block. It could aggravate the pain in the short term and the pain in her leg was better dealt with by reverting to rocking the knees and rolling along the spine for several minutes.

The BackBlock was the most effective way of decompressing the central core impaction at the lumbo-sacral level and I asked Sally to visualise this happening: the spine lengthening as the legs pulled the pelvis off the bottom of L5. She should also visualise the right facet pulling apart and dispersing its swelling, even if this gave her some pain running deep into the right buttock as she did it.

Two weeks after I had first seen her, Sally telephoned to say that she had been painfree in the leg and the back for over a week. She was using the

BackBlock (plus curl ups) routinely but had not spontaneously taken to using it in the early and middle part of the day as some people do. Instead she was using it at the end of the day when her back was looser and this way she felt freer when she woke up. Most importantly, Sally was using the Block and feeling its benefits. This is significant because I know when people get addicted to it, their days of back trouble are nearly over.

When she called I instructed her in the use of a tennis ball to mobilise the old problem with the L5 facet. She was to place it under the joint and lower her weight onto it. She was then told to 'worry' the joint by moving minutely back and forth over the painful spot.

Fifth treatment

This final treatment took place several weeks after I first saw Sally. She now had very little backpain and no trouble at all from her leg. It was time to implement her own final stage exercises—the Cobra and Pose of the Child— to mobilise the still-gummy facet and encourage cartilage regrowth.

The pronounced arching hang of the Cobra exercise particularly mobilises the lumbo-sacral facets. Although it forcibly compresses the joint surfaces and causes a typically sharp pain, the close-packed position disperses residual swelling and subjects the joint surfaces to much higher pressures. Sally found the exercise quite tolerable and could feel her spine dropping down cog by cog into a deeper hollow.

I explained to Sally that this latest routine was always to come at the end of her other exercises because it requires the spine to be maximally supple. She should repeat the 'long' forward hangs of the Cobra two or three times, followed by the antidote posture of the Child, and then she should do several see-sawing movements. These should be done slowly at first and then faster as she improved.

4 The acute locked back

An acute locked back occurs when the spine slips slightly out of joint at one of the facets.

WHAT IS AN ACUTE LOCKED BACK?

An acute locked back is when an unguarded movement causes an agonising jolt of pain like a high voltage current to shoot through your back. The pain always strikes at the beginning of a movement, like a bolt from the blue, and leaves you bent over rigid and unable to straighten .

Usually the pain catches you so badly you cannot stir. You cannot go forwards or backwards, or put one foot after the other. It is a real crisis. Often it makes the knees buckle so you collapse to the floor and an injection of pethidine may be needed before you can be moved. It is always a very frightening experience, and often unforgettable many years later.

There are an infinite number of minor ways you can suffer an attack like this. You can do it turning over in bed, getting out of a car, pulling your chair out, bending forward to pick up a toothbrush, lifting a bale of wool. One patient did it zipping up a ball dress. Common to all is the unexpectedness and a certain lack of exertion. In fact, absence of effort and preparedness for what you were about to do, seem to play a key part.

As a therapist, I find acute facet locking one of the most daunting conditions to treat. At the time of the crisis patients are in extremis; they are loath to move and almost hysterically fearful of doing anything that might cause another jolt of pain.

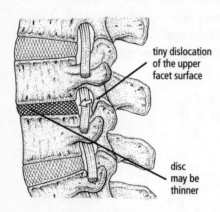

tiny dislocation of the upper facet surface

disc may be thinner

Figure 4.1 Sometimes an unguarded movement, with the tummy unbraced, can cause a facet to jump imperceptibly out of joint.

90

Long after the original episode has passed they remain fearful of it happening again and often feel their back is never the same again (indeed some feel their *life* is never the same again).

Over the years, many opinions have been put forward as to what goes wrong. Although acute locked back feels as if something has slipped out, it is most definitly *not* a slipped disc. However there is never any objective evidence to explain exactly what has happened. There is nothing to see on the X-rays or other forms of scanning, and the neurological assessment is usually clear. Yet there is a fellow human cast down and immobilised, often on the floor as if caught in a freeze frame, and literally rigid with pain.

One popular explanation is the jamming of a meniscoid inclusion (a tiny wedge of cartilage from the margins of the facet joint) between the two joint surfaces, which sends all the muscles of the spine into a gust of protective spasm. A similar, more plausible, explanation points to the nipping of the sensitive folds of synovial membrane between the facet joint surfaces.

I believe the main cause of facet locking is a momentary lapse of spinal coordination, causing a facet at the back of the spine to slip slightly out of joint. Almost before a movement has begun, the spine is caught unawares and one facet moves slightly out of alignment. If pinching of the synovial lining does happen, I suspect it is only part of the wider picture of the vertebra slipping askew and the joint jamming.

The degree of movement is infinitesimal so it is never possible to take a picture and see any joint dislocation. But the actual slip is not the problem. The reaction is: an instantaneous and massive protective response from the muscles which takes your breath away as they lock up the spine.

A joint being 'out' anywhere else in the body does not arouse the same defence. (We have all experienced a wonky knee when our kneecap temporarily mistracks.) However the spine's heavy responsibilities for

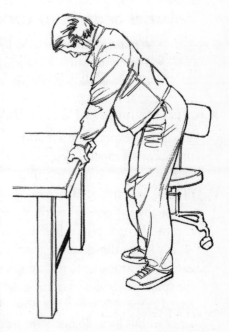

Figure 4.2 When you are stricken by a locked facet it can be impossible to move.

structural support and protection of its fragile festoonery of nerves inside make it keenly alert to any threat to its integrity.

When facet locking happens in the neck it is relatively easy to manipulate back into position. The neck's slender accessibility makes it much easier than the low back where bulky protective spasm quickly sets in, making it difficult to pull the segments apart. If you are lucky to get to an osteopath/chiropractor/physiotherapist soon enough, a small high speed manipulative thrust, with its characteristic popping sound, can break the jamming of the joint and reposition the vertebra correctly.

These are the wonder cures you occasionally hear of. The technique momentarily gaps the joint open and lets it slot back together in proper apposition. If it is successful, the joint immediately rides freely again, and you can walk away on air with none of your former pain. Any residual muscle spasm will be gone by the next day.

More usually though, by the time you get to a practitioner the stiffness of the muscles is so well established it stops the joint being physically opened. Attempting manipulation at this stage only makes matters worse. It alarms the patient (because it hurts) and causes the protective hold of the muscles to intensify.

CAUSES OF AN ACUTE LOCKED BACK

- A natural 'window of weakness' early in a bend
- Segmental stiffness predisposes to facet locking
- Muscle weakness contributes to facet locking

A natural 'window of weakness' early in a bend

All spines experience a natural vulnerability on bending until they get themselves properly braced. I believe that facet locking occurs when the spine is caught momentarily ill-prepared as it passes through a fleeting 'window of weakness' in the early part of range.

Bracing happens when the muscles at the back and front of the abdomen contract in unison to stiffen the spine. They create a valuable tensile strength which keeps the spinal segments secure until they can be passed into the care of the strong system of muscles and ligaments running down the back of the spine. These then pay out slowly and lower the spine forward like a mechanical crane. However, the powerful long back muscles and the 'posterior ligamentous lock' do not come into their own until the spine is well forward into a hoop when at last they generate sufficient tension to make the spine safe.

Up until this time the spine passes through an unsprung phase when it must rely on the tummy muscles to tense the abdomen and slightly hump the spine to get it across the wobbly part. This slight tensing and humping in preparation for bending plays a subtle but invaluable role in putting the important multifidus and transversus abdominus muscles in a better position to act. They control the tipping of the segment by being intimately involved in the gapping apart of the facets to allow the segments to go forward.

But even the slightest delay of one or other partner in the co-contraction can cause a hiccup in the movement. When the spine starts to move before both systems are ready, it is caught off guard and minutely disjoints somewhere in the column at one of its facets. The threat this poses to the spine causes a massive protective response from the muscles which jam the slipping facet before it can go any further. This is the reaction which brings you to your knees.

A locking incident often happens when people are recovering from a viral illness. Generalised debility is the most likely explanation, when the reflexes are dulled and the tummy muscles (in particular) cannot generate a quick enough response to keep the spine supported.

Facet locking can also happen a day or so after some form of serious exertion such as laying paving stones, cutting timber or digging in the garden. In these circumstances, it is probably the overactivity of the long back muscles and their residual raised tone which disturbs the natural harmony of the two deeper groups working underneath. The story is always the same: your back has been feeling stiff for a day or so and it was harder than usual to keep the tummy pulled in. Then some minor incident—almost too incidental to be taken seriously—catches you when you least expect it and brings you down.

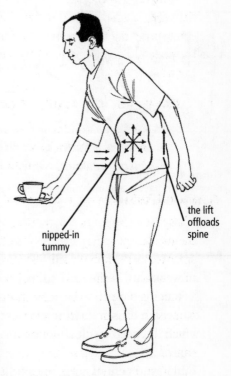

nipped-in tummy

the lift offloads spine

Figure 4.3 When bending forward, a tight tummy offloads the spine and tenses the spinal links.

Segmental stiffness predisposes to facet locking

Segmental stiffness, even when benign and painless, can predispose your back to locking if the intervertebral disc between the two segments has already lost its umph.

One of the specific roles of the multifidus muscle (with its willing helper the 'muscular' ligamentum flavum on the other side of the facet) is to pre-tense the intervertebral disc at each lumbar level. As soon as your spine starts to move, the disc should be as tense and plump as possible to prevent any wobble of the vertebra. If the disc has already lost fluid and the intra-discal pressure has dropped, it is much harder for the facet muscles to get the disc primed. Thus a spine already in line to develop symptoms from a stiff segment is also more likely to suffer a facet locking incident.

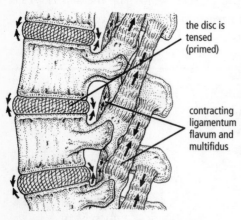

the disc is tensed (primed)

contracting ligamentum flavum and multifidus

Figure 4.4 A vital action in early bending is ligamentum flavum and multifidus priming the disc to prevent wobble.

If the disc has already dropped in height and the other ligaments holding the segment in place have become slack, the segment is additionally vulnerable. The bone against bone locking of the facets (which provides a more basic tier of stability) is not specific enough to prevent minute movement of a vertebra and the facet can slip slightly askew unless the volitional muscular hold (the tummy) is compensating well. In fluke circumstances, an ill-prepared tummy can bring the whole lot down.

Muscle weakness contributes to facet locking

Longstanding segmental stiffness often makes the muscles weak. When a segment is too stiff to be active the small muscles which work it have less to do, which causes them to atrophy. This particularly applies to multifidus which lies deep inside, right on the back of the facets, acting as their special protector.

In its moment of need, multifidus may find when its segment goes to slip it is not up to the task of keeping its joint under control. This is particularly important when a back has been suffering underlying trouble for some time. When there is low grade inflammation of a facet, there is evidence to suggest that multifidus 'deliberately' under-performs to spare the irritable joint excessive compression. Although this might be for the prevailing comfort of the inflamed facet in the short term, in the long term it leaves the facet without the muscular control to compensate for other inefficiencies. A problem facet is wide open to a future locking episode.

Apart from this automatic inhibition, primary weakness of muscles can also cause facet locking. General indolence or unfitness can so impair our streamlined coordination that the tummy and back muscles fail to cooperate simultaneously in holding the spine supported. In a brief blip of control they perform out of sync, also making it difficult for the deeper intrinsics to come in at just the right time. If they fail to hump the back in its imperceptible first few degrees of bending, and the two important deep muscles cannot develop an optimal line of pull, the fundamental unit at the centre of the motion segment—the disc—does not get primed properly, and the segment can slip.

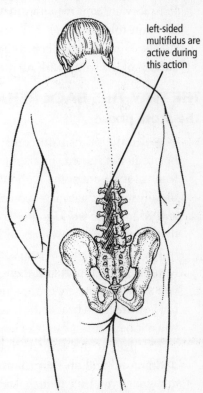

left-sided multifidus are active during this action

As a first cause, a weak tummy is easy to blame because it affects so many of us. Most of us harbour a lax 'underbelly'. Weakness here creates a sloppy hydraulic sack which is less efficient at forcing the spine skywards. With a weaker up-thrusting force within the abdominal cavity and failure to round the back, there is a reduced tensile strength between the spinal links, leaving them more susceptible to jostling about when the spine moves forward.

Women are particularly susceptible to this in late pregnancy and early motherhood. When the tummy is stretched and weak and the ligaments still soft from the pregnancy hormones, it is easy for the muscle system to be less prepared for spinal action. This can also happen to any of us suffering

Figure 4.5 As we bend down to the left, left-sided multifidus hangs onto the tail of the vertebra and steadies it, preventing it swinging across to the right.

from exhaustion, unfitness or recent obesity. Getting up after an illness it is also possible to suffer a locking incident, probably because of generalised weakness. Food poisoning and the flu are also commonly mentioned as predisposing conditions.

The relative weakness of multifidus in its role of preventing sideways twist of a vertebra may also contribute to facet locking. Since all functional bending movements incorporate a twisting component (unlike robots which have an up–down and left–right action only) multifidus is like David against Goliath in steadying the torque of the heavy trunk above. Even though the available range of segmental rotation is a few degrees only, multifidus (acting one-sidedly) is the only muscle which directly controls its vertebra. It does so at the very beginning of range by hanging on to its tail and preventing it from going both forward and twisting sideways. (Iliocostalis, another intrinsic muscle, also controls the vertebra twisting but only deeper into the forward bend.) All the other muscles controlling spinal rotation are in large sheets on the surface of the trunk with no direct attachment to the spine.

THE WAY THIS BACK BEHAVES
The acute phase

The electric jolt of pain comes at the beginning of a movement—almost before it has started. In a split second there is an ominous sort of 'uh oh' feeling, as if your spine is about to do something it shouldn't. The action is usually inconsequential—you can be leaning forward to pick up a coffee cup and your whole world stops. Apart from the suddenness, you are speechless that something so trivial could have brought you undone.

The sudden clench of pain completely takes your strength away. You clutch furniture for support and then, with your hands sliding down your thighs, you slither helplessly to the floor. There at least you are more comfortable but you are like a beached whale and nobody can move you. If you are alone when it happens, it can take hours to crawl to the telephone to call for help.

The pain at this stage can alternate between a cramp hovering in the background and an excruciating jolt whenever you move. If you need to move a leg you have to inch it across using a sideways heel–toe action on the floor. If you attempt to lift the leg or jerk in any way the pain will zap you again and leave you gasping.

What causes the pain?

The grabs of pain in the acute phase come from the muscles locking up the whole spine to trap the individual joint. They jump instantaneously into a high-pitched clench whenever they sense the joint trying to move. It is strange that the protective response causes so much pain. The muscle contraction stops the mini-dislocation going any further but it also prevents the joint disengaging and repositioning correctly. The muscles keep on keeping on, like a dog with a bone, and they are a major part of the problem.

The intense compression of the joint while it is still out of kilter sends out the usual alarm signals of any traumatically twisted joint. The back does not let you off as lightly as a twisted ankle does, probably because of the complexity of the workings inside the back and the relative size of the tiny joint compared to the bulk of the muscles guarding it. Until they are satisfied they can relax, they stay guarding the joint, keeping it out of action and locked away in the machinery of the whole spine.

The special mechanical receptors in the capsule let the brain know the joint is locked under pressure. They do so the instant the joint freezes and repeat the message every time there is even so much as a flicker from the muscles. Several hours later, a different sort of constant low-grade pain creeps in from the stimulation of the chemical receptors in the joint capsule. They register the build-up of toxins in the tissues, both from the original capsule-tearing damage and the stagnant circulation through the capsule. As the concentration of toxins rises the protective spasm increases, which intensifies the hold on the joint and the pain coming from it.

The muscle spasm itself can cause a similar type of constant pain. When blood must be squeezed through tonically contracted fibres, the metabolic waste products cannot get away. As their concentration rises, their irritation of the free nerve endings in the joint's tissues is read as pain. Cramping muscles also experience another type of pain from lack of oxygen (anoxia). The over-working muscles cannot get sufficient fresh supplies through, creating a typical tired pain with peaking pin-prick twinges after being still for too long.

Pain begets more spasm which begets more pain. Unless you start moving and get the joint active the cycle intensifies. Accordingly, reducing the muscle spasm and getting early movement is important early in the treatment regimen. When you have just been struck down however, any therapy seems a long way off. At the time, the pain seems to come from everywhere and the back feels rock hard.

At this stage, the best course of action is an intra-muscular injection of pethidine (a strong pain-killer) and a muscle relaxant such as Valium as well. The first priority is to get you off the floor and into bed and the quicker a doctor is called the better. For your future rehabilitation you need to get over the incapacity stage as soon as possible.

If the first attack is not handled properly you may never get over it, either physically or emotionally. Many people with ongoing troubles claim their problem started with an incident like this which was never properly resolved. Twenty or thirty years later they can remember every detail and they tell you their back has never been right since.

The sub-acute phase

Within a matter of a few days, the crisis of the acute condition should pass. With resting in bed and proper medication the muscle spasm relaxes and it is easier to move. Your own attitude makes a big difference here. The more fearful and tense you are the more you hold things up. Keeping calm and deliberately making your spine move again helps break through the stiffness and relieves the pressure on the jammed joint. The more anxious you are, the slower this resolution is.

As the muscles relax, it becomes easier to lift your bottom off the bed although it is still painful to turn over. Slowly the guarding reaction loses intensity and the back softens its armour-plated hold. There are no crippling jolts of pain if you move slowly. Unless you make a sudden jerking movement or sneeze or cough you will be able to get up, although it is difficult doing something complicated like getting out of bed.

Slowly the broad expanse of pain retracts to a localised area of soreness and it is easier to pinpoint the focus of the trouble. By this stage your back usually feels bruised and fragile, as if it has been through an ordeal. Even though it is weak, it is ready to get moving.

The chronic phase

In its chronic phase this problem behaves the same as facet joint arthropathy (see Chapter 3). When the blanket of protective spasm lifts, the joint underneath often emerges as dysfunctional. It needs to be mobilised as soon as possible and brought up to par with the rest of the joints, otherwise the problem becomes chronic and continues off and on indefinitely.

When the damaged facet is slow getting going the protective muscle spasm hangs around and the condition worsens. There is shrinkage of the joint capsule as a legacy of the scar tissue formation but in a seemingly contradictory way, the capsule may also be left weak. Microscopic scarring cobbles the joint and pinches it tight, which leaves it stiff, but the original renting of the joint capsule and the weakness of the local muscles around it leave it weaker and easier to re-injure in future.

Taken to its extreme, the facet joint may eventually become unstable (see Chapter 6). This condition brings with it a conundrum for the joint's management. How do you strengthen the stiff and inelastic joint capsule when its very stiffness may be the only thing holding it together? This is the problem facing all facet instabilities, and it is not an easy one to deal with. Better therefore to handle it early on—after the first facet locking episode—so you never have to deal with the difficult end.

The aim is to get the joint going early to lessen the scarring. Even if your problem is longstanding (when you fear that loosening the joint will make it pop out again), the joint must, nevertheless, be mobilised, while making sure to cover the new-found freedom with improved power of the segmental muscles. The most effective way of doing this is by intrinsic exercises, unfurling the trunk off the end of a table, but an easier version is simply touching the toes.

If the intrinsic power of the segment is not restored quickly you are left with a back you keep hurting with twisting movement. You bend down to help an elderly lady with her luggage and you feel the familiar tweak as you overtax the weak facet. By next day your back has stiffened and developed its familiar lateral 'S' bend with one hip protruding. It feels tighter and caught up on one side and you keep digging your fingers in to find relief.

People often seek treatment at this point because they can do less and less before they tweak the weak facet again and it takes progressively longer each time to recover. Whereas it used to be two or three days in bed now it takes ten and you are barely over one attack before the next one comes along. One episode appears to merge with the next.

WHAT YOU CAN DO ABOUT IT
The aims of self treatment for an acute locked back

The immediate aim in treating an acute locked back is to quell the alarm, so at the very least you can move your limbs without pain and turn over in bed. After the crisis has passed, it is important to deal with the joint sprain, and then bind up the problem joint with good muscle support so it does not happen time and again.

Getting the muscle spasm to relax is best achieved by muscle relaxant drugs and strong painkillers, often administered by injection. As soon as the drugs start to work, the spine must be moved to lessen the clench of the muscles and release the joint. This is started as soon as possible—taking one leg up at a time, and rocking the knees to the chest, fingers interlaced around the knees—and repeated innumerable times throughout the day. It usually takes less than 24 hours to be able to move your legs in bed comfortably and to sit up without difficulty.

The sooner the next phase can be commenced, the faster the problem resolves. Both relaxation of muscle spasm and the return of normal movement of the injured joint are achieved by gentle curling up exercises. Working the tummy muscles hard relaxes the spasm of the long back muscles and encourages normal gliding and hinging of the locked vertebra. As soon as the joint starts moving, the trapped engorgement disperses and the pain eases dramatically. In many respects, the treatment at this stage is similar to the chronic phase of facet arthropathy, although there is a greater emphasis on re-educating the muscles to control the wrenched facet.

The final stage of treatment is devoted almost entirely to improving both the strength and the coordination of the various muscles influencing the injured joint. The strength of the deep muscles compensates for the traumatic stretching of the capsule and ensures the joint is not left susceptible to repeated lockings. At the same time, stretching of the long back muscles, particularly into full bending movements, inhibits their tendency to overact which automatically keeps the deeper ones weak. The bending exercises (toe touches) also relieve the general stiffness of the back.

A typical treatment for acute locked back

(See Chapter 7 for description of all exercises and the correct way to do them.)

Purpose: Relieve muscle spasm, decompress the jammed facet joint

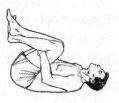

Rocking knees to the chest (60 seconds)

Rest, knees crooked resting together (30 seconds)

Rocking knees to the chest

Rest

Rocking knees to the chest

Rest

Rocking knees to the chest

Rest

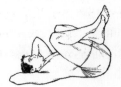

Reverse curl ups (five times)

Rest

Reverse curl ups

Rest

Medication: intramuscular pethidine followed by muscle relaxants and anti-inflammatories (NSAIDS) administered only by your doctor. Rest in bed. Repeat treatment regimen every 30 minutes or less often if you are sleepy from the drugs. When commencing the rocking exercise, always lift one leg to your chest at a time. The legs are very heavy and if you try hauling both up together you will jerk your back and set off another seizure of pain.

For how long? If you can begin the medication soon enough, you may be able to start the sub-acute treatment by the next morning.

A typical treatment for sub-acute locked back

Purpose: Relieve muscle spasm, strengthen tummy, start mobilising the jammed facet joint

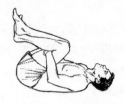

Rocking knees to the chest (for 60 seconds)
Curl ups (five times)
Rest (for 30 seconds)

Rocking knees to the chest
Curl ups
Rest

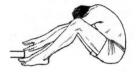

Rocking knees to the chest
Curl ups
Rest

Rocking knees to the chest
Curl ups
Rest

Curl ups (ten times)
Rest

Curl ups
Rest

Rest after each session with your lower legs supported on pillows. Repeat three times daily but do not hurry. Always expect the first one or two curl ups to be more painful and always take care to curl up without hunching your shoulders. If you come up with a straight trunk you will hurt your back.

It is actually possible to be painfree after your first successful session of curl ups. If it is too painful for you to curl up, you must revert to the acute regimen for another session. You must stay on this sub-acute regimen until you are largely painfree doing the curl ups and there are no sudden seizures of pain with unguarded movement. This usually takes two to three days to achieve.

A typical treatment for chronic locked back

Purpose: Decompress spine, mobilise facet joint, strengthen multifidus muscle to
control the facet, strengthen tummy

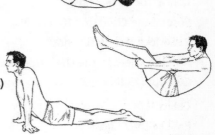

Rocking knees to chest (for 60 seconds)
Pivoting on vertebra (for 15 seconds)

Cobra (for 10 seconds)
Pose of the Child (for 10 seconds)
BackBlock (for 60 seconds)
Rocking knees to chest (for 60 seconds)
Curl ups (15 times)

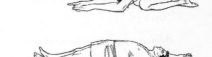

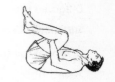

Cobra
Pose of the child
BackBlock
Rocking knees to the chest
Curl ups

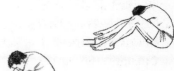

Squatting (30 seconds)
Toe touches (three times down and up)
Diagonal toe touches (four to bad side: one to good)

Squatting
Toe touches
Diagonal toe touches

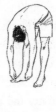

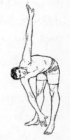

Your back will feel generally sore and
fragile when caught off guard but there is
no sense it will let you down. It will feel
stiff and sore after sitting in one position
for too long, and tired and achey if you
have been on your feet for too long.
When this happens you should lie down
and gently rock your knees to your chest
until the pain goes. You may progress to
the next regimen when your back is
largely painfree.

A typical treatment for sub-chronic locked back

Purpose: Mobilise problem facet joint, strengthen the facet muslces to stop it jumping out of joint again, improve the coordination of the spine.

Tennis ball (for 15 seconds)

Cobra (for 10 seconds)
Pose of the Child (for 10 seconds)
BackBlock (for 60 seconds)
Rocking knees to the chest (for 30 seconds)
Curl ups (15 times)

Cobra
Pose of the Child
BackBlock
Rocking knees to the chest
Curl ups

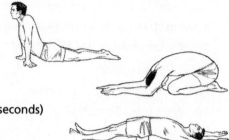
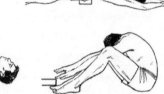

Floor twists (two to bad side: one to good side)
Squatting (for 30 seconds)

Diagonal toe touches (four bounces bad side: one good side)
Squatting

Diagonal toe touches
Squatting

Intrinsics (12–15 times)
Rocking knees to chest
Rolling along spine
Curl ups

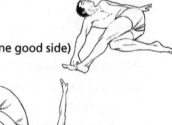

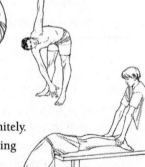

The entire treatment program need not be continued indefinitely. After the episode has faded you need only persevere with using the tennis ball BackBlock and diagonal toe touches twice a week. However, you should always squat throughout the day whenever your back feels tired and clenched. You will retain a sensitivity and a weakness of the damaged facet for a long time, so you cannot afford to completely forget about maintenance exercises. Remember, when doing the diagonal toe touches, you will find bending to the bad side always more restricted than bending the other way.

A CASE HISTORY OF AN ACUTE LOCKED BACK

Sam is our 54-year-old farm manager, who had been a shearer in his youth and suffered one episode of sciatica. His back had not troubled him since, although he would be stiff getting upright after shoeing horses or using a chainsaw. He had recently put on some weight and was having trouble doing up the top button on his trousers.

Sam was in the process of loading wool bales from the floor of the shearing shed. He was using two sharply pointed bale hooks to save him bending deeply, but as he went to lift, one corner fouled on a box on the floor and caught him at an odd angle.

He felt a sharp pull in the side of his spine and thought he had pulled a muscle. He got the bale rolling across the floor to the open doorway and the waiting truck but could not lift it on. Within two or three minutes he was very uncomfortable and had to sit down on the step.

Sam wasn't incapacitated immediately by the pain but he felt something go and a sense of breathtaking tightness lock up in his back. He had difficulty walking away and got back to his house to lie down on the floor. Although he tried to keep going for the rest of the day it was harder and harder to remain upright.

By the time I saw him mid-afternoon he was nearly bent double on his back porch leaning on a long stick like a shepherd's crook. The bottom of the stick kept breaking off from the force of him trying to hold himself upright, with his hands grasping the top end. Each time the stick broke, the shock reverberating through his body nearly brought him down. He barely had the breath to speak and looked a strong man sadly incapacitated.

Sam was not brought to the ground in the first instant by the back locking up, so his signs and symptoms were slightly atypical. His case demonstrates the wide variability in the presentation of all back problems, which should not confuse the main picture. In this case, stoicism probably kept him going.

Sam took some anti-inflammatory tablets in preparation for his first treatment at the end of that day. He was aware of the complications of these drugs, with their noxious effect on the digestive system, and the plan was to continue them for only a few days. We had no muscle relaxants at hand, so made do with what we had.

First treatment

When I arrived to treat Sam he was slightly more relaxed and breathing more freely, but his back was no less painful; he was bent like a banana and could not straighten or bend deeper. His spine also deviated slightly to the right and the muscles on the right side of the spine in particular were visibly in spasm.

The main object of treatment at the outset was to get his back relaxed enough to palpate and to establish at which level the jammed facet joint was. I chose to treat him on the floor where he had spent most of the afternoon. He got down on his back and I put two pillows under his head.

We began with the usual gentle rocking of knees to the chest to try to stretch out the clench of the muscles. It was a slow job and we had to start cautiously. First one knee then the other was lifted, with my help, and then with fingers interlaced around knees, the gentle oscillations began.

This was continued for about two minutes at a time, and repeated twice more. It soon became obvious the focus of the pain was on the left of his spine, and higher than the oscillations were reaching. We then altered the technique and brought Sam's knees up higher on his chest so that he was curled up more into a ball. Although it took slightly more effort, Sam said it felt more as if it was prising open the painful joint. It was uncomfortable but unthreatening.

I then turned Sam over to treat his back from the other side. He lay on a pile of pillows on the floor to temporarily safeguard his bentness. On the first attempt to turn him over he jerked his spine and we lost some of the ground we'd gained. Another two lots of knee rocking were necessary to get us back to where we were.

Since the jammed facet was higher up in the spine, probably at the L3–L4 level on the left, I did not follow the loosening techniques with the curl ups I use with lower back problems. Instead I went for the modified form used in just these circumstances, curl ups in reverse, where Sam's head stayed on the pillow with his hands linked behind the neck, and he brought his knees up to meet his chin. He repeated as many as possible, which was only about eight or ten times. Afterwards, he found it easier to let each leg down to the floor.

With Sam as relaxed as possible in the prone position, I mobilised the joint by slowly rocking his pelvis from side to side. I did this by rotating the hips towards me with my fingers hooked around the iliac crest (the hip bone) and letting the elastic recoil of the muscles take it back the other way.

Using counter-pressure with my left thumb against the side of each spinous process in turn, I established that L3 was stiff. At the neurocentral core this segment moved as one block with the vertebra below. I made no attempt to palpate down onto the injured facet between L3 and L4, because I knew it would be too uncomfortable, and the reactive spasm would flick me off the joint.

After doing the hip rotation for several minutes I asked Sam to join in, swinging his hips rhythmically from left to right by rotating his lower abdomen.

He took care to keep it gentle and rhythmic because if he got too enthusiastic he would get a another jab of pain.

Sam turned over onto his back again by rolling himself sideways off the pillows like a log, and I put two pillows under his head. After another session of rocking his knees, I instructed Sam to keep doing this for as much of the evening as possible, and then go for a walk. I specifically asked him to walk tall, deliberately trying to off-load his back and take the pressure off the jammed link. It was also important to let his hips swing, keeping up a steady but careful pace.

An hour and a half later I was astonished to see Sam poke his head around our kitchen door. He had walked from his place to ours, a distance of less than a kilometre. He was standing straight and looking chirpy, with virtually no pain.

This was an unusually good result, but in my experience it is preferable not to have a quantum leap like this first off because it is impossible to match with successive treatments. Although patients feel on the right track, there are fewer ups and downs and mood swings if the progress is more slow and steady.

Sam was instructed to do more rocking of the knees to the chest and reverse curl ups on the floor before going to bed that night and to repeat the knees to the chest exercise in bed on waking in the morning.

Second treatment

Sam had been warned he would stiffen up by morning so he was not unduly worried when it occurred. He was more concerned that his back felt sore, as if he had been kicked by a horse. He did a long session of rocking his knees followed by another at noon, and I saw him again that evening.

By then he was standing straighter, but still moving stiffly and wary of unguarded movement. He had arrived at the point where I inherit most of my patients. It is rare for me to see people so early on, most having been through the first part of the crisis alone when they have simply stayed in bed for a week to ten days.

Treatment began with knee rocking exercises and then I put him onto his stomach again. Once prone, he was comfortable with just one pillow under his tummy. In the flatter position I repeated the hips rolling technique, with counter-pressure against L3. After 60 seconds I removed the pillow and asked him to continue the hip swinging in the flatter position. After another 60 seconds I asked him to rest on his forearms in the position of a Sphinx, and I took over the sideways rolling of the pelvis. It took several seconds for the spine to let down, as if cog by cog. At first it was painful and the tummy tried to hold the spine and prevent it sagging forward. Sam needed to be persuaded to relax his tummy and buttocks to let the spine sink.

He rested flat for a minute or two and then the rotating Sphinx was done twice more. As he continued tipping his pelvis, the motion gradually became more undulating, spreading right throughout his body, which is always a good sign. I then asked Sam to roll over on his back and after briefly rocking the knees, I asked him to roll back and forth along the length of his spine, pivoting on the painful spot. Sam was instructed to do these two last exercises again before going to bed.

Third treatment

The third treatment was on the fifth day. Sam was quite sore after the second treatment but had discontinued taking the anti-inflammatory drugs because they made him feel sick. He no longer had the sense of his back grabbing on sudden movement and opted to feel sore rather than keep taking the pills.

His posture was now straight and he could also bend forward, albeit somewhat stiffly. It must be stressed that Sam had arrived at this point much sooner than most. More often, the first and second treatments need to be repeated for up to four to five days with as long as ten days before the Sphinx exercise can be started. The blanket cover of anti-inflammatories administered so early obviously speeded up progress.

By the third treatment Sam's back was sufficiently relaxed (as shown by his ability to bend forward) that I felt it was time to investigate the facet problem itself. Palpating with my thumbs about 1.5 cm to the side of the spine between the knobs of the third and fourth spinous process I could feel the soft squashy mass of the left L3–L4 facet.

The capsule was not tense (it would have been earlier when locked by the muscle spasm) but it was sore and slightly puffy. I mobilised it briefly to disperse the residual fluid and then asked him to repeat his spinal rolling exercises for 60 seconds to help loosen the neurocentral core of the segment as well.

I showed Sam how to mobilise the facet by lying on his back with the knees bent and placing a tennis ball under the sore joint. As he lowered his full weight down onto the ball he felt the familiar grab of pain as the muscles attempted to guard the joint. By relaxing and sinking on to the ball he could avoid the sharp pain, but he was quite uncomfortable.

Sam was advised to use the tennis ball sparingly (no more than twice a week for less than 30 seconds each time). Its purpose was primarily to disperse swelling rather than overcome stiffness of the joint and in this regard it differed from the intense mobilising pressures needed for chronic degeneration of a facet, where you might use it three times a week.

Fourth treatment

This treatment took place seven days after the locking incident. By this stage there was very little pain from the back although it felt stiff in the mornings and after being in one position for too long. The third lumbar segment was still less mobile on forward gliding palpation and the left facet was stiff on deep probing to the end of range of the joint.

Sam had continued his full home routine for twenty minutes every evening and was back to working on the farm. To complete his treatment however, it was critically important to restore the strength and coordination of the muscles of his spine. The intrinsic muscles had to be re-educated to gain better segmental control of the problem level and also to switch off the overactive long back muscles.

Leaving these muscles as they were would leave the injured link unprotected. It would also cause ongoing disharmony of spinal mechanics which would increase the risk of hurting the back again. To strengthen multifidus which specifically controls the facet joints, we went straight to the strenuous intrinsics exercises. With Sam lying face down with his hips at the edge of the table and me securing his legs on the table, he lowered his upper body to the floor. The return journey to horizontal he did in a segmental unfurling fashion, from the base of his spine up, with his head coming up last.

For a strong man Sam found this unusually difficult to do. Partly because of the bulk of his chest and shoulders, he felt weak across his lower back. At the start he had difficulty with the humping action and found it hard doing more than ten exercises. After a brief rest he managed a further ten.

Because Sam had a demanding physical job he did not need to continue this table exercise on a regular basis. He did however need to regularly do the toe-touching exercises to improve the automatic control of his bending. These are a less arduous form of intrinsics but require greater coordination. They selectively recruit the deep muscles over the superficial ones and require deliberate control from the tummy muscles to keep the spine braced.

As well as the normal toe touches, Sam was also taught the diagonal form (with the stance wide) to re-educate the strength of multifidus working one-sidedly. Because the locking mishap occurred on the left, it was important to target the muscle fibres on the left of the spine. Bending forward and taking the right hand past the left ankle and unfurling diagonally back to vertical did this. Compared to the same movement on the other side (the left hand to right ankle) the movement was stiffer, which is usually the case. Sam was asked to do the exercise more often to the left than the right in a ratio of four to one, and to repeat it at various intervals through the day. He should do five or six at a time at least four times each day, especially after alighting from a vehicle. This would keep his spine segmentally strong.

5 The prolapsed (slipped) disc

A prolapsed or slipped disc occurs when the vitality of the disc breaks down and the back wall bulges where it perishes.

WHAT IS A PROLAPSED DISC?

A slipped disc is a bulge in the back wall of the disc which fails to disappear when the pressure comes off. The condition needs explaining because for years it has carried the can as the main perpetrator of mischief in backs. In the 1930s, discs were said to be the chief cause of back trouble, and this limited view of what goes wrong has held sway almost to the present day.

When anything sudden happened it was thought that a disc had popped out of spinal alignment—like a saucer slipping out of a stack—and was pinching a nearby spinal nerve. With a more generalised low grade backache, the diagnosis would perhaps run to the discs disintegrating or collapsing. (Only lately has facet joint arthritis come to the fore.)

Sometimes a disc wall does bulge, but by modern estimates fewer than 5 per cent of back problems are caused by this. True disc prolapse involves a localised bulging of the wall, when the degenerated nucleus loses cohesion with the breakdown process and squirts off-centre. The pain is not so much from the disc (because the disc is like fingernail and hardly has a nerve supply), but from other pain-sensitive structures outside which are offended by the bulge.

If the bulge obtrudes straight out the

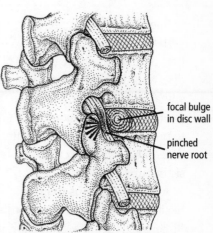

focal bulge in disc wall

pinched nerve root

Figure 5.1 As a disc loses vitality, a focal bulge can appear where the back wall collects greatest stress.

111

back of the disc (a posterior bulge) it may push into the bundle of nerves hanging down from the cord and cause 'cauda equina symptoms'. These can include deep central backpain, impotence, disturbances of bowel control and micturition (passing urine) and/or saddle anaesthesia. If the wall bulges towards the diagonal back corner of a disc (a postero-lateral bulge) it may squash the spinal nerve and cause sciatic pain down the leg together with numbness, pins and needles and weakness of muscle power in the calf or foot.

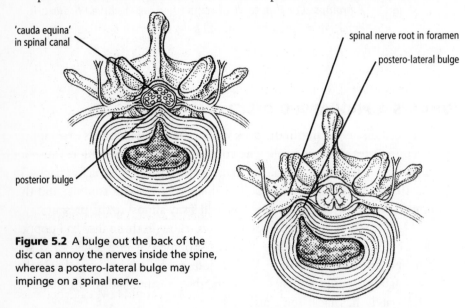

'cauda equina' in spinal canal

spinal nerve root in foramen

postero-lateral bulge

posterior bulge

Figure 5.2 A bulge out the back of the disc can annoy the nerves inside the spine, whereas a postero-lateral bulge may impinge on a spinal nerve.

Spontaneous disc prolapse, where there was nothing previously wrong with the disc, is a non-event. When prolapse does come about, I believe it is part of a much wider picture of breakdown—when the weakening of the disc wall develops over a long period of time. It never happens when the spinal segment is healthy, when the discs are far less likely than the vertebrae to break or split. (Laboratory studies subjecting the spines of young cadavers to progressive loading eventually caused the bones to rupture rather than the discs. The vertebrae crumbled into a bony rubble while the discs remained sitting up as good as new.)

A disc never slips to cripple you with one blinding movement. In their healthy state discs are extraordinarily strong and never dislodge with one ill-considered move. Discs are very superior segmental connectors. They make powerfully bendable fibrous unions between the vertebrae and are so strong they are one of the main agents keeping the segments together. Believe me, nothing slips freely anywhere.

Sometimes a facet joint can jump very slightly out of joint (see Chapter 4) but a disc wall simply bulges (prolapses) and in some cases bursts (fenestrates) spewing out its contents—the denourished nucleus—into the canal cavity where it may float about or wrap itself around the spinal nerve root (sequestrates). Disastrous as this sounds, the nuclear material is eventually absorbed by the blood stream, although if it is very degenerated, the body may set up an auto-immune response in the meantime which irritates the nerve.

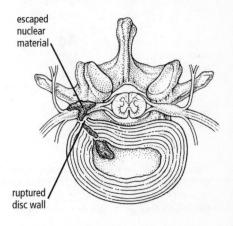

escaped nuclear material

ruptured disc wall

Figure 5.3 Sometimes compression on a sick disc can cause the wall to rupture and spew out its nucleus which wraps around the nerve root.

Perhaps the pure expressiveness of the term 'slipped' has captured the imagination of patients and specialists alike and slowed the pace of change. When a back is devastatingly and persistently brought down, the very word conjures images of something bad happening; of something slipping off centre and jamming the works, even though the spinal mechanics are far too sophisticated for anything so crude to occur. It is ironic that so much for so long has been put down to such an unlikely cause; that this rare condition could have obtained such wide currency, as to be almost inversely proportional to its true incidence.

In truth, there are many instances of disc prolapse—but as a source of backpain it is extremely rare. This has only been provable in recent years with the advance of 'magnetic resonance imaging' (MRI) techniques. Large cross-sections of the population *not suffering from backpain* were scanned (without the radiation hazard of X-ray myelography) to see what the general run-of-the-mill back looked like inside. What emerged was an astonishing one in five people under the age of 60 with ruptured discs who did not know they had a problem. This figure rose to an equally astonishing one in three people over the age of 60 with detectable ruptured discs of the spine—also without symptoms. Nearly 80 per cent of those scanned had bulges. Clearly, bulging or ruptured discs are not the mischief makers they were always held to be.

I believe a disc bulges when other problems of the motion segment cause muscle spasm to set in. Most of the surrounding structures are highly pain-sensitive and can easily make the muscles go on guard when they are inflamed. If the protective response continues indefinitely, it compresses the segment and eventually makes the disc wall distend. The tonic vertical clench of the muscles, particularly across the problem level, slowly squeezes the disc out, where its bulging adds to the general congestion.

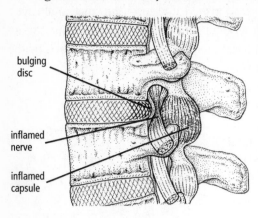

bulging disc

inflamed nerve

inflamed capsule

Figure 5.4 When everything inside the segment is bloated and inflamed, the disc is the easiest structure to section out, although its removal may make the facet capsule pucker more.

Healthy discs never do this. They briefly broaden by a millimetre or two as they take weight but this is not the same as the segment jamming and causing a tense balloon of weakness in the wall. Healthy discs are extremely resilient and never bulge or burst at whim. The story of slipping a disc by moving awkwardly and developing a sudden pain down the leg is not one of acute disc prolapse. There must always be a history of pre-existing breakdown—even if it was silent and gave no symptoms along the way.

True disc sciatica usually has a slow lead-up over several years, manifesting in the early days as the grumbling backache of segmental stiffness (see Chapter 2). Eventually it becomes something different, as the original backpain disappears and a new type of pain develops down the leg.

Diagnostic techniques

Discs have always been difficult to talk about with conviction because they are difficult to see. Because disc material is not radio-opaque it is not possible to get a clear picture on X-ray. To find out if a disc was protruding into the spinal cord (in the spinal canal) or the spinal nerve (in the intervertebral exit canal), a radio-opaque dye was injected into the space around the cord and its investments, then the patient tilted this way and that to make it trickle around the discs. Afterwards an X-ray was taken to reveal the discs' outline. The procedure is called a myelogram.

Fortunately this very clumsy and unpleasant procedure (which often left the patient with headaches for days but much more seriously sometimes caused 'arachnoiditis'—a longstanding inflammation of the tissue coverings of the spinal cord) has been completely superseded, first by CT scans and then by MRI (magnetic resonance imaging). Although MRI in particular is very expensive, it shows increasingly clear (almost 3D) images of soft tissues and bone alike, making it much easier to interpret the state of play of all spinal structures, not just the discs.

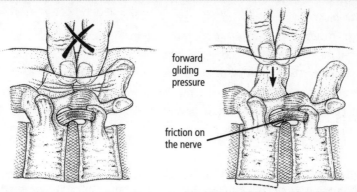

Figure 5.5 The disc is at the front of the spine, so the thumbs cannot feel what is going on.

Figure 5.6 Indirect pressure on a disc through the spinous process can provoke leg pain by causing friction of the bulge against the nerve.

It is impossible for people like me to feel the discs with our hands because they are around the front of the spine and far out of reach of our probings. It is only possible to feel the state of the neurocentral core by palpating it through the vertebra's backward tail (the spinous process). Although there may be a typically 'gummy' feeling from the back when there is a tense disc bulge, this may be difficult to pick up. Sometimes however, the slight palpatory pressures disturb a bulge and provoke pain further afield, probably by the swollen wall rubbing against the nerve root.

If minimal pressure brings on a cramping leg pain, it spells out a high irritability of the nerve—although it is important to exclude facet involvement, rather than disc. This is done by feeling 1–2 cm laterally from the centre, over the facets.

Because it is impossible to feel the disc we must rely on objective signs to show if the spinal nerve root is under duress. They are all called 'neurological signs' and they indicate the degree of irritability of the nerve and the extent to which it has stopped working. The straight leg raise test (SLR) consists of raising the leg to a right angle and not allowing the knee to bend. By increasing the tension on the nerve roots you can tell if one is inflamed. If there is a marked nerve inflammation the leg barely gets off the bed before it exacerbates the leg pain. Other signs of nerve involvement are dulled or absent reflexes (behind the ankle and below the knee), numbness of the skin on the leg and loss of muscle power. It is confusing that severe inflammation of a facet joint gives almost the same signs (see Chapter 3). I believe you can only conclude that symptoms are caused by disc prolapse if there are disturbances of bowel and bladder function (which a facet cannot cause).

You can only be absolutely sure it is the disc if there is nothing wrong with the facet. All too often in practice a patient arrives at my clinic with the diagnosis of a 'disc in need of surgery', showing all the signs and symptoms of a nerve in distress. And yet the most perfunctory mobilisation of the facet at the same level fixes the problem in a matter of days. With this the case, it is hard to believe the disc was the chief problem in the first place.

True disc prolapse is one of the hardest spinal conditions to fix conservatively—but it will respond. Once the nucleus is out of the centre it is difficult to get back (it is often described as getting toothpaste back into a tube). The only hope is mobilising the segment as a whole to release it from compression. The loosening relieves the pressure on the bulge and allows the disc to keep more of its fluid. It also restores a better circulation to the area which reduces the inflammation caused by so many swollen structures inside the segment, all pressing and chafing up against one another, the disc but one.

Even with stark evidence of disc prolapse on a CT or MRI scan it can be nothing short of miraculous how well a case like this can do. If the crimped spinal segment can be made to move normally with the rest of the spine, even the most menacing leg pain will go away. However, once a nerve root has been badly inflamed it retains a lowered threshold long afterwards. For many months and even years it is super-sensitive and very susceptible to flare-ups, especially after sitting. With even the slightest recurrence of muscle spasm, or if the circulation becomes sluggish for other reasons, the old familiar leg cramp can start up.

Disc surgery

The fact that the whole 'metabolic climate' inside an inflamed segment contributes to the irritation of a nerve root may explain why removing a disc with surgery is so often unsuccessful. Some figures estimate that 50 per cent of operations for a slipped disc leave the patient worse or at least no better. Removing the disc may not be removing the problem; it may be worsening it. If indeed the facet is the main source of pain, wholesale disc removal obliterates the disc space and brings more pressure to bear on the facets. After the operation the leg pain is much worse—which is very depressing after all you have been through. No sooner are you upright than all your symptoms return, as bad as they ever were. Sometimes you hear of repeat surgery two or three weeks later to operate on another level.

However, many back operations are extremely successful. In the past, a more radical procedure called a laminectomy was performed which removed the entire disc (by picking away at it with scalpel and pliers, like tearing away pieces of fingernail) and then part of the bony ring above and below the nerve was removed. Sometimes a spinal fusion would then be performed during the same operation to deal with the instability created by destroying the fibrous union. The fusion was performed either by packing out the empty disc space with bone chips (usually taken from the hip bone) or inserting two large screws through the facet joints.

More recently, spinal surgery has become less invasive (and less upsetting to the beautiful spinal mechanics when the spine has to get going). A micro-discectomy is a much finer operation and smacks less of removing the tyre and letting the wheel run along on the rim. This procedure is carried out through a tiny cut in the skin and takes as little disc as possible (virtually the bulge only). With a smaller wound and less cutting, the scar formation is also kept to a minimum.

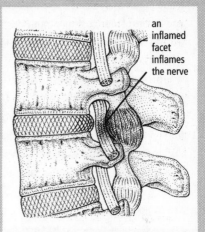

an inflamed facet inflames the nerve

Figure 5.7 If both disc and facet are tensely swollen, the changeable leg symptoms are more likely to come from the facet. The facet's rich blood supply makes it more mercurial.

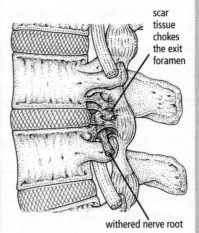

scar tissue chokes the exit foramen

withered nerve root

Figure 5.8 Scar tissue is like living undergrowth which invades the machinery of the segment.

Apart from the essentials of skill, the most successful surgeons repair the cut made in the thoraco-lumbar fascia before they close up. This means the vertebral segments retain their ability to clench vertically in preparation for spinal activity (which ultimately helps avoid instability problems). It also pays to keep the blood and oozing fluids to a minimum during the operation, and mop up as much as possible before closing the wound. Many surgeons demand the resumption of normal activity as soon as possible after a disc is removed. (The most successful surgeon I ever worked with, would not discharge his patients until they could touch their toes—usually ten days after surgery.) Early activity disperses old blood and lymph collected in the tissues, so fewer adhesions clag the works, and it gets the working parts of the spine moving again.

The more selective surgeons have strict guidelines, and operate only if there is evidence of the nerves in the saddle area and legs not working properly. Pain alone is no reason for opening a back and removing a disc. It is too emotive and too subjective. And besides, there are many other spinal disorders which can produce similar pain. It is too awful if the disc is removed and the pain is still there—and it happens all the time.

CAUSES OF A PROLAPSED DISC

- Pre-existing breakdown alters the properties of the nucleus and weakens the disc wall
- Bending and lifting stress breaks down the back wall of the disc

Pre-existing breakdown alters the properties of the nucleus and weakens the disc wall

Discs are shock absorbers and are meant to bulge. In their healthy state, the girth of each one swells imperceptibly as we transfer support from leg to leg during routine weight-bearing activity. As compression passes downwards through the spine, forces are transmitted outwards in all directions via the fluid of the nucleus. Through the mechanics of an hydraulic sack, compression is converted to a springing buoyancy which gives the spinal links their tensile strength and prevents the column juddering as we make contact with the ground.

As the spine sinks and springs with movement there is a synchronised to-and-fro exchange of energy. This passes between the briefly distorting nucleus and a moment later, the stretching mesh of the disc wall as it accommodates the force. When the wall nears its limits, its elastic recoil bounces this 'energy' back to the nucleus causing it to puff up from within.

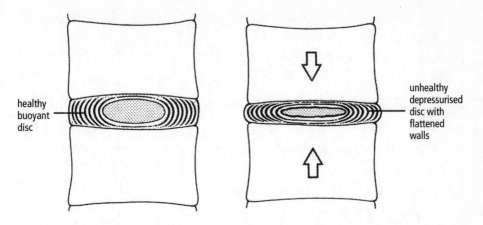

Figure 5.9 As the disc loses vitality, it becomes drier and unresponsive and cannot spring-load its vertebra during movement.

This sublime dynamic uses the tension of the disc walls to off-load the weight of the spine bearing down from above and gives us spring in our step.

The transfer of energy works well while the nucleus and the disc wall are in peak condition. As long as the nucleus retains its proper viscosity and the wall keeps its tensile strength, a disc can dissipate on–off compression indefinitely. But early breakdown of either the facets or the disc—and protective muscle spasm which is too energetic—can change everything. Stiffness at the front of the spinal segment and facet arthritis at the back, can eventually lead to disc prolapse by destroying the viability of the disc.

The muscle spasm is often the first key; even a fleeting problem can become permanent if protective muscle spasm never goes away. The clamp of the muscles keeps the segment compressed in a vice which hinders the dynamics of the on-off compression. As the muscle clamp and the compression persist, the disc starts to bulge around its full circumference, like the spare tyre of the Michelin man. From this mild and reversible fattening the disc can start to break down.

As the disc dries out and the nucleus becomes more viscid, it is more easily deformed under pressure. Instead of being a tightly contained ball of fluid at the centre of the disc, the nucleus loses cohesion and spreads out when compressed. As it squirts this way and that with different activities of the spine, the nucleus bumps up against the internal layers of the disc wall, its only means of constraint. Over time, the battering against the interior walls amounts to trauma of the inner layers and they start to perish.

Activities which increase the pressure inside the disc, accelerate its breakdown from within. With generalised slumped sitting for example, when the pressure within the discs is raised, more force is directed towards the back wall of the disc. But with bending, which always involves some twist, the force is directed to the left- or right-hand back corner of the disc.

Bending and lifting stress breaks down the back wall of the disc

When the nucleus is on the run, ever-present bending of the spine has dire consequences. The intra-discal pressure is great when the spine bends forward.

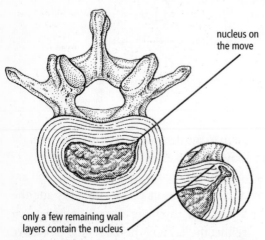

nucleus on
the move

only a few remaining wall
layers contain the nucleus

Figure 5.10 With torsional lifting strains, multiple fibre breakage at one point on the disc wall can form a small nick, which the runaway nucleus burrows into.

If there is a degree of twist as well, the pressure is even greater, because the muscle effort increases the clamping-down pressure on the disc. If the twisting action is always in the same direction the nucleus damages the same part of the inner wall and breaks it up, strand by strand, like elastic fibres in a corset perishing at the points of greatest wear.

Strenuous lifting can be the last straw. It places enormous stresses upon the spine, particularly the lowermost discs. It raises the intra-discal pressures to unparalleled heights and as more fibres break in the same spot, a radial split opens up in the wall from the inside out. With more lifting and more pressure, the squirting nucleus burrows its way into the opening and prises it apart as it makes tracks towards the periphery. Eventually the whole wall may split open, disgorging its nucleus into the spinal canal.

Intensifying the breakdown

Rupture of the disc happens faster if the weight being lifted is held out from the body or if the lifting is heavy work—both of which increase the internal pressure of the disc. It also happens faster if you bend over using a large twisting element to lift. The disengaging of the facets as the segment goes forward makes the disc even more vulnerable to torsional strain and the alternating layers in the wall tend to separate, making circumferential tears in the outer zones. This appears to happen more readily in kidney-shaped discs, where the hard outer wall buckles around the sharper corners of the disc. With marked internal derangement of a disc, a radial split can meet up with a circumferential one and the nucleus can squeeze through many parts of the wall.

The combination of the internal squirting pressure of the nucleus and the rotatory strains on the wall means the disc is most likely to break down at the points corresponding to 5 and 7 o'clock on the clock face. This explains the preponderance of postero-lateral disc bulges. The predominance of right postero-lateral discs bulges (as opposed to left) is probably explained by the dominance of right-handedness in the community. Additional pressure is exerted on the right side of the disc by the muscles of the right side of the trunk and the right arm.

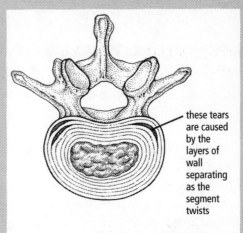

these tears are caused by the layers of wall separating as the segment twists

Figure 5.11 Circumferential tears tend to be more common in the acute-angled corners of kidney-shaped disc walls.

In a good example of Murphy's Law, the two points at the diagonal back corners of the disc are exactly where the sciatic nerve roots make their way out of the spine, having branched off the spinal cord higher up. They travel down

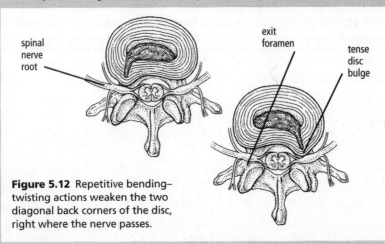

spinal nerve root

exit foramen

tense disc bulge

Figure 5.12 Repetitive bending–twisting actions weaken the two diagonal back corners of the disc, right where the nerve passes.

inside the canal as multiple strands and then exit via the left and right inter-vertebral foramen at their designated level.

With a posterior protrusion the nerve root can be blighted inside the central spinal canal, but a postero-lateral bulge can irritate the nerve inside the exit canal (or foramen). There is less room in the foramen than the central canal and the nerve can get doubly assaulted. It can be squashed up against the far wall while at the same time being stretched over the back of the bulge, like squeezing past the fat lady in the bus.

Not surprisingly, slipped discs are often brought on by strong physical work. Heavy twisting–lifting actions are the worst: digging with a long-handled shovel or repetitive bending to move boxes from the same height. Nurses are particularly prone to back trouble, though not always discogenic. Bad lifting techniques can weaken the disc wall but the disc must already be in trouble for the nucleus to prolapse.

Most commonly nurses get a bad back when they save a patient from falling. This may make the disc wall rupture but it is more likely to strain a dormant stiff link in the spine (either of the front or back compartment) which may or may not have been causing symptoms beforehand.

THE WAY THIS BACK BEHAVES
Acute disc prolapse

Sciatic pain usually creeps up over several days after hurting your back. You can usually recall exactly what you did although it is rare to feel your back go at the time. You probably feel a slight strain in your back, with a momentary deep pain inside which passes off quickly. You might hurt your back with an awkward lifting action, where the object is unwieldy rather than unliftable. You may be hauling up one end of a sofa for example, and attempting to push it across the floor, when a corner snags. The difficult wrestling which follows is often the last straw and there is a sharp feeling of strain in your back. It becomes more sore and tight over the next few days, and then the pain down the leg starts.

The overwhelming feature is a painful tension deep in your buttock and down the leg which develops into a nasty cramp-like pain. In the beginning it feels like a pulled muscle or a tightly pulled string in the leg. It often originates in your buttock and moves down into the thigh, missing out on the knee and reappearing in the calf. You can usually locate a trigger point deep in your buttock by digging in through the layers of muscle with your fingertips, and for some reason, pressure here relieves the pain in the leg.

The nerve may be so inflamed and sensitive to stretch you cannot even get your heel to the floor when standing. Your back often acquires a lateral bend or sciatic scoliosis to relieve the tension of the nerve root and the whole back has a painful crippled appearance. Sometimes the sciatic scoliosis can be so pronounced, with the hips out one side and the shoulders the other, that you look as if you won't fit through a doorway. From the rear view the spine looks completely hunched over and weak. As well as its lateral 'S' bends it will have a lumbar hump instead of a hollow. The buttock of the bad side can be flat and wasted, making a continuous line with the rounded low back. Both spinal deformities are protective mechanisms to minimise the tension on the inflamed nerve root.

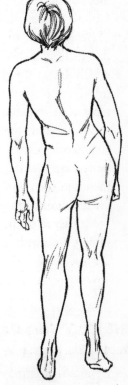

If you have to stand, you rest your weight on your toe and keep the knee bent to avoid stretching the nerve, and the leg often shakes uncontrollably. Walking is reduced to a pathetic hobble. Every time you take a step forward there is a dreadful, mind-numbing pain down the leg like a jagged, red-hot spear through the tissues (which the textbooks describe as 'lancinating' leg pain). Bending forward is just as impossible. As you attempt to go over, there is a crippling pain down your leg and the spine slews off more into its wind-swept deformity to avoid the stretch.

Figure 5.13 True disc prolapse is a pathetic sight. When standing, you cannot put your heel to the ground and walking is reduced to a hobble because you cannot stretch the nerve to take the leg forward.

Sitting is often unbearable because the bunching down of the spine increases the pressure on the disc and hence the tension on the nerve. After a few seconds the pain can be so bad you have to get up and lean on something to hang your leg to take the weight off. The pain can be just as unbearable after a few minutes of standing, when the pressure on the disc increases to a crescendo of cramping pain. (You hear of people on their way to being admitted to hospital having to lie down on the floor of the elevator to find relief.) The most comfortable position is lying on your side in the foetal position with a pillow between the knees.

What causes the acute pain?

The backpain of acute disc prolapse is probably caused by the stretching of the disc walls and the pain genesis here is not dissimilar to that of stretching a stiff disc (see Chapter 2). The pressure on the localised bulge stimulates globular mechanical receptors between the fibres which manifests as a deep uncomfortable pain inside your back which is not relieved by the pressure of hands.

However the disc itself is not particularly pain sensitive. Only the outer one-third of the wall has a nerve supply which explains why smaller bulges, which are so common, are invariably painless. These can be thought of as full-thickness bulges where the intact inner layers of the disc wall absorb most of the pressure of the nucleus discharging laterally. They save the more sensitive outer layers of the disc wall from the immediate force of the nucleus.

Once a degraded nucleus is on the move, it acts like a wedge which penetrates a small nick in the innermost walls and spreads it wider as it moves to the periphery. As it gets closer, with fewer remaining layers left to contain it, the tension on the disc wall becomes immense, further fuelled by the pressure of the muscle spasm. (This may explain why a problem disc often bursts with a loud popping sound when the surgeon's scalpel breaches it at surgery and the nucleus flies metres across the room.)

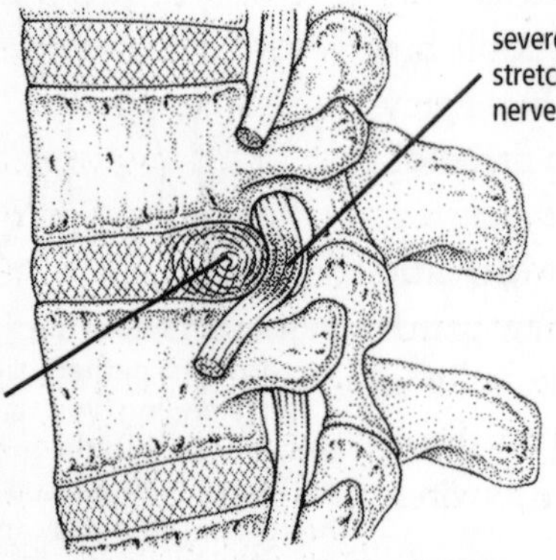

As the condition becomes more serious the old familiar back pain disappears as the leg pain comes on. This may be caused by the nucleus spontaneously bursting right through the outer wall. This relieves the pressure on the wall but it may create other problems. By this stage, the nucleus may be a brownish colour (indicating it is degraded and toxic) and this can chemically irritate the nerve root—especially if the nerve has already been sensitised by pressure.

severely stretched nerve root

tense focal bulge

Figure 5.14 With large disc prolapse, the tension of the nerve stretched over the bulge causes more pain than the nerve simply being squashed.

It is thought that stretching a nerve root causes more trouble than mere pressure. After all, we know from leaning on our funny bone at the elbow that nerves tolerate pressure quite well. It may temporarily lose conduction as the arm goes to sleep, and it is unpleasant and pins-and-needly while it wakes up again, but there is never raging pain. Pulling a nerve taut, thus subjecting it to friction as well as tension (as it twangs and rubs past other structures) is a much greater irritant. Thus a lesser bulge which does not stretch the nerve will not be painful, explaining why such a high percentage of the population have disc bulges with no accompanying pain.

The first effect of pressure (and tension) on the nerve root is to restrict circulation. Fresh blood is prevented from squeezing through to the affected part, and stale blood damming up cannot flush the products of metabolism away. Both circumstances irritate free nerve endings in the local tissues which register another tier of discomfort from the problem area.

Remember, the inflammatory reaction does not apply to the disc itself because it is virtually bloodless. Rather, it applies to all the other red and swollen tissues clustering around the swollen disc and adding to the engorgement. This racks up the muscle spasm across the segment to another level, which adds more compression and makes everything bulge even more— including the disc. Everything becomes more inflamed and squashed together in a confined space.

When the nerve is under pressure and stretched as well, there is friction between the tightly stretched nerve and its own protective sheath. The physical chafing between the two hyperaemic (blood-congested) surfaces causes much more pain as the inflammation of the nerve intensifies. Clear fluid weeps from the raw and angry surfaces, such as you see from a burn of the skin, and the pain becomes unspeakably bad. If you could look inside you would see the nerve grotesquely red and swollen and the surrounding tissues swimming in fluid. This is the metabolic climate which causes agonising pain in the leg and which is very difficult to settle conservatively.

The disc, as the least bloody structure of the segment, is not a bad choice for surgical excision if the problem gets that bad. When everything is locked by irreversibly bloated congestion, this highly pressurised but inert component is the easiest to define and section out. It is a quick and effective way of decompressing a segment when all conservative methods have failed, despite the ill-effects this may have upon the future function of the spine.

Chronic disc prolapse

By this stage the bulge is no longer much in evidence, although the disc is under duress of a different kind. In the chronic phase the internal machinery of the segment struggles with the after-effects of inflammation, and the pain may be coming from several different problems at the same time. For example there may be symptoms of chronic segmental stiffness (see Chapter 2) and facet arthropathy (see Chapter 3) as well as chronic tethering, or fibrosis, of the once-inflamed nerve root.

As a legacy of the previous pitch of inflammation, the weeping exudate from the nerve gradually solidifies into thickened strands of scar tissue. This forms a matted mess, gluing the nerve to its sheath and other structures nearby, including the wall of the exit canal. Dry, whitish adhesions permeate everything, creating a choking collar which gradually strangles the nerve. This is called 'root sleeve fibrosis'.

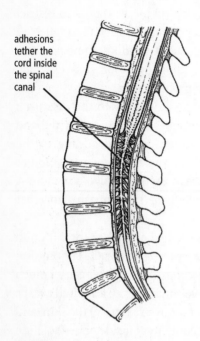

adhesions tether the cord inside the spinal canal

The tethering stops the nerve pulling and retracting freely through the bony tube as the moving leg exerts traction on it. A dense undergrowth of adhesions dominates, often binding the nerve down to the back of the disc. The nerve is often much thinner than it should be because it has been under tension for so long.

Your leg can feel like a rigid extension of your back. It cannot bend freely at the hip to sit, nor make a step forward to walk, without taking your back along with it. This causes a typical waddling gait, where the low back rotates in a bottom-twisting fashion instead of your leg angling cleanly backwards and forwards in the hip socket. Your back is stiff, with different pains according to what you do, and the pain down your leg comes and goes, depending on how much tension you put on the nerve.

Figure 5.15 Dural tethering occurs when a myriad strands of scar tissue bind the cord to the internal canal, just like Gulliver's hairs pegging his head to the ground.

Sometimes the spinal cord is tethered to the inside of the canal wall. When sitting, the back is not free to slump and there is a dull pulling sensation which spreads high into your back and down into your buttock and thigh. This is called 'dural tethering'. The sitting stretches the spinal cord and tugs it where it adheres to the wall, causing a deep gasping pain which can extend to the shoulder blades. Sometimes you can almost feel the tightness inside the spine bowing you forward.

If the tethering is restricted to the nerve root in the exit canal, most of the symptoms are in the leg. With sitting, the buttock wants to come forward to lessen the acute angle at the hip, and the knee bends automatically when you attempt to straighten your leg. After a time, sitting may bring on other symptoms, like numbness of the heel, or a pain under the foot. But the tight dull pain in your thigh will always be worst because the slumped posture causes traction on the nerve root where it is glued to the foramen. Long after all other symptoms have gone away, a lengthy car trip or aeroplane flight can bring on a pain which you have not felt for years.

Apart from the cobbled-up leg and the difficulty sitting, there may be other subtle signs of the nerve not working properly. There can be a low-grade wasting of the muscles of the bad side. The buttock can look flat and withered, as can the calf, where the muscle has less tone and is floppy. There can also be less obvious signs, like the arch of the foot slowly dropping which causes the forefoot to splay out, sometimes making you feel your foot is too big for your shoe. You may notice that certain actions are weaker: you cannot stand on your toe or push off with that foot. When you walk, your leg feels heavier and more difficult to control and you have to haul it up when you take a step.

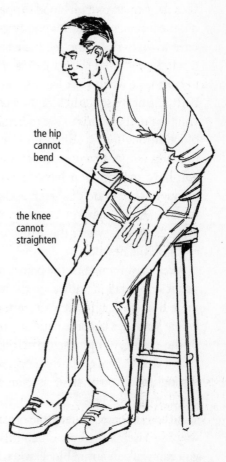

the hip cannot bend

the knee cannot straighten

Figure 5.16 A tethered nerve cannot pull free of the exit canal (like a strand of cooked spaghetti clinging to the pot), as the stretching leg puts tension on the nerve.

What causes the chronic pain?

Aggressive tension strains on the nerve, such as you might get kicking a football, can cause a localised inflammatory reaction right at the point where the nerve is bound down. Instead of the nerve pulling loose out of its exit canal, like a strand of cooked spaghetti, it is barely free to budge. The wrench may break a few adhesions and cause a small bleed in the otherwise whitish tissues, which then goes on to create more scarring and increases the cobbling effect. In the meantime there is more of the familiar pain in your leg, as the nerve is sensitised by the local inflammatory reaction.

Beyond a certain point, the invasive proliferation of adhesions may cause symptoms of 'vertebral stenosis'—internal narrowing of the spinal canal—because the nerve's own blood supply is hampered by the living junk crowding out the foramen. With this condition you feel pain in the legs whenever they have work to do. You often have to stop and sit down after walking a short distance, and even sooner going up hills or steps.

Normally, when your leg muscles have to pump vigorously to move your body, the nerve sucks in blood to keep it relaying messages back and forth to your brain. If conditions are too cramped the nerve cannot puff up to get the blood through. As it suffers anoxia (lack of oxygen) your legs get more and more leaden, until a dreadful cramping pain locks them up completely and you have to stop. You have to rest by bending over or squatting, which broadens the inside diameter of the spinal canal and gives relief by letting more blood through. You can also get vertebral stenosis with facet arthropathy (see Chapter 3) where the arthritic bulk of the facet joint creates a similar effect on the nerve.

After a few moments, the pain eases and you feel more comfortable. When you resume walking however, the pain starts up sooner and you have to rest more quickly. Each time you start, you travel shorter and shorter distances before your legs become painfully burdensome again and slow you to a halt. By the end of your journey, you feel you have barely started before you must stop. (This feature of shorter and shorter distances covered between respites distinguishes spinal stenosis pain from the cramping leg pains caused by circulatory problems.)

Although there is a tangible organic reason for the legs locking up in this way, it is fascinating how much this can change from day to day. Some days you can walk an entire block and the next you can barely get down the path to the street. The variable in the equation is the degree of muscle spasm in your back. When present to any degree it compresses the segment and further inhibits the blood getting through. In this regard, anxiety and tension also have a role to play because they influence the degree of tone in the muscles. If you are particularly tired or uptight, your legs will be harder to move and you will have the familiar wading-through-treacle feeling over the smallest distances. Other days, for what seems no good reason, you could almost be walking on air.

WHAT YOU CAN DO ABOUT IT
The aims of self treatment of a prolapsed disc

In the acute stage of disc prolapse, the overriding concern is to gap open the back of the lumbar vertebrae to take the pressure off the bulge. This is achieved by rocking the knees to the chest, but benefits will be short-lived unless the muscle spasm can also be relaxed. This will not happen unless the inflammation of the soft tissues is dealt with. Medication prescribed by your doctor is necessary on both counts (NSAIDs [anti-inflammatories] and muscle relaxants). Doing early reverse curl ups, even when there is severe sciatica, will also help ease the muscle spasm in the back.

As soon as the vascular engorgement is on the move and the inflammation of the nerve has started to settle, it is important to seek more permanent separation of the segments. This is where both the BackBlock regimen and the squatting exercises come in. Both bring about a suction effect which drags fluid into the discs and puffs them up. At the same time, the more strenuous curl ups raise the intra-abdominal pressure, which lessens the bearing down pressure on the discs.

In the chronic phase of disc prolapse the emphasis is both on stabilising and stretching. Sometimes segmental instability is waiting in the wings, brought on by lower intradiscal pressure and weakening of the disc wall. Both toe touches and diagonal toe touches will suck fluid into the discs as well as strengthen the deep intrinsic muscles across the interspaces. The diagonal toe touches and the diagonal floor twists also work to stretch adhesions in the exit canal which may be a legacy of past inflammation. The nerve root may be tethered to other structures nearby, and the rhythmic stretch and release of the nerve, pulling with the bending, helps persuade it free. At this stage, rotatory spinal movements also loosen the diagonal lattice of the disc wall, which frees it up to imbibe more fluid.

A typical treatment for acute prolapsed disc

See Chapter 7 for descriptions of all exercises and the correct way to do them.

Purpose: Relieve muscle spasm, gap the back of the vertebrae to relieve the pressure on the bulge

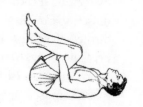

Rocking knees to the chest (60 seconds)

Rest, lower legs on pillow support (30 seconds)
_____

Rocking knees to the chest

Rest
_____

Rocking knees to the chest

Rest
_____

Rocking knees to chest

Rest
_____

Rocking knees to the chest

Rest
_____

Rocking knees to chest

Rest
_____

Medication. Rest most of the time in bed with the lower legs supported on a stool or pile of pillows, hips and knees at 90 degrees. Repeat the knees rocking and reverse curl ups at least every 30 minutes.

For how long? You can progress to the sub-acute regimen when the leg pain is no longer constant.

A typical treatment for sub-acute prolapsed disc

Purpose: Relieve muscle spasm, decompress spine to rehydrate the disc, strengthen tummy to lift weight off the disc

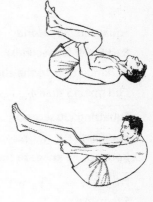

Rocking knees to the chest (60 seconds)
Rolling along the spine (15–30 seconds)
Reverse curl ups (five times)
Squatting (30 seconds)

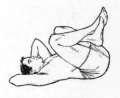

Rocking knees to the chest
Rolling along the spine
Reverse curl ups
Squatting

BackBlock (60 seconds)
Rocking knees to the chest (30 seconds)
Reverse curl ups (15 times)
Squatting

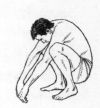

Treatment sessions should be early in the morning and afternoon, followed by rest, with the lower legs supported, for 20 minutes. When you are up and about, you should avoid lengthy periods of sitting and standing still, and try to have two short walks per day (less than 15 minutes), walking briskly and lightly on your feet. It is best to have two short walks per day and spend the rest of the time lying down.

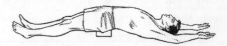

A typical treatment for chronic prolapsed disc

Purpose: Decompress the base of the spine, stretch adhesions, restore coordination between the tummy and the two groups of back muscles

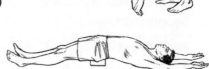

Squatting (30 seconds)
BackBlock (60 seconds)
Rocking knees to the chest (30 seconds)
Curl ups (15 times)
———
Squatting (30 seconds)
BackBlock
Rocking the knees to the chest
Curl ups
———

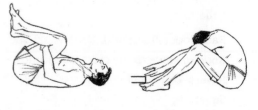

Squatting
BackBlock
Rocking the knees to the chest
Curl ups
———
Squatting
Floor twists (two to bad side: one to good)
———

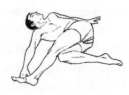

Squatting
Floor twists
———
Diagonal toe touches (three times) (four to bad side:
    one to good)
Squatting

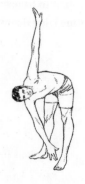

Repeat three times per week. If the curl ups cause pain down the leg, change them to reverse curl ups. Otherwise, you should only have leg pain after lengthy periods of sitting or travelling. If you do, you must revert to the sub-acute stage regimen.

A CASE HISTORY OF A PROLAPSED (SLIPPED) DISC

Graham is a 44-year-old public servant who had been a super-fit triathlete when his back broke down. At the time he had been running up to 80 km per week and cycling 50 km. He had had his first bout of trouble many years earlier when he felt a twinge in the centre of his low back doing warm-up twisting exercises before a run. He wore a back brace (made of hard plastic) for six months until he got 'fed up' and discarded it, but his back was never the same again. Thereafter he felt much less flexible (he could only bend forward far enough for his fingers to reach just below the knees), and he noticed his back had lost its natural lumbar hollow.

Graham's main back crisis did not come until eight years after the first episode, when he walked 10 km with a backpack. Afterwards his back was niggling and stiff but he didn't hit rock bottom until a few weeks later when he travelled in a car with small bucket seats forcing him to sit with his knees under his chin. In his own mind this was when he felt his disc 'slip'. He could barely stand when he got out of the car, with severe pain in the central low back and down the back of both legs to the ankles. The leg pain lasted three or four weeks during which time he was also unable to sit or stand. He continued working by lying on the floor in his office with his computer on a low coffee table.

I did not see Graham while he passed through this period, and in a sense he got through the initial acute phase on his own by lying down most of the time. I first saw him when he was well into the sub-acute phase. Leg pain was no longer a problem but he had a severe cramping pain across his low back (and slightly to the right) which would rise to a crescendo of stiffness spreading into the buttocks if he sat or stood for too long.

On initial examination, straight leg raising (which tests the irritability of the lower nerve roots) of his right leg was reduced to 45 degrees and caused a pain in the left side of his back. There was no muscle weakness or disturbances of sensation. CT scans showed a minor disc bulge at the L4–L5 level and at the L5–S1 a 'large right sided posterior disc herniation compressing the thecal sack and impinging on the S1 nerve root'. I believed he was getting most of his backpain from a large central bulge pressing into the posterior longitudinal ligament, although this may have distended laterally earlier and collected both S1 nerve roots (thus causing the leg pain). His forward bending was restricted to fingertips to the knees and the spine veered tightly to the right as he went over.

Graham's back looked sinewy and uncompromising. It had an unusually cobbled appearance, with kinks and bumps of the vertebral links, like a barnacled anchor chain. (I assumed this was the legacy of hundreds of miles of running on hard surfaces.) The segmental irregularity was particularly obvious as he bent forward, with those above L4 kyphosed and prominent, and L5 deeply recessed. All the way up to the base of his neck, the vertebrae deviated one way and the other, with flattened or recessed patches in his otherwise kyphosed thoracic spine. In short, his spine looked a mess, with a marked thoracic kyphosis atop a too flat lumbar spine giving him a slightly hunched look.

To me, his back illustrated the whole sequence of spinal breakdown from the niggly, gripey back pain of segmental stiffness in the early days, to disc prolapse and segmental instability as he stood before me. Apart from the reduced straight leg raise and the evidence of disc herniation on the CT scan, the clearest indication of disc herniation was the back's gummy resistance to bending forward and its stubborn unresponsiveness to manual treatment. The typical twisting movement in the base of the spine as he bent forward was evidence of segmental instability. (Incidentally, this did not show up as such a fluid twist in the early days when the spine was almost rigid. Then it presented more as a list to the right as he went over.)

First treatment

On palpation, the entire spine felt as stiff as it looked. L5 was particularly immobile, with L1 and L2 less so. Treatment was started by rocking Graham's knees to his chest for several minutes to relax the spine enough for me to feel inside. Even then, L5 was difficult to get at and did not 'melt' in the way a stiff segment does. It retained a rubbery end-of-range feel, although mobilising a stiff right sacro-iliac joint and T10 and T11 at the base of the thoracic kyphosis did cause them to thaw. In fact, Graham's back retained such a board-like rigidity that I soon changed from mobilising the segments manually to spinal rolling and reverse curl ups, which were more successful at breaking up the stiffness. He was encouraged to do all three loosening exercises at home as much as he could until the next visit.

Second treatment

As I might have predicted, Graham's early signs of 'lightness' in the back did not last more than a few hours. It was obvious from the resilience of his symptoms that he would be more suited to a 'softly, softly' approach of consistent disimpaction, rather than anything hard hitting. Like all true prolapse problems, the bulge was the culmination of years of trouble. It would not disappear until the pressure came off the disc, and the weakness in the wall could regenerate in its usual stately manner. Intensive 'hands on' treatment would simply make it sore. Treatments with me were therefore weeks, sometimes months, apart.

Graham's back needed a sustained program of lengthwise decompression, both to restore segmental mobility and to re-establish better spinal alignment. In particular, he needed to open out the hunched kyphotic posture which caused constant 'turning moment' strain of the upper body tipping forward on the lumbo-sacral junction. He also needed to have a proper functioning lordosis in his low back restored, which had not been there since he had worn the brace years before. Both corrections would reduce the neurocentral compression of the L5 segment.

He had been aware during his triathalon training how his cycling posture played havoc with his back. Often he could barely get off his bike, let alone stand up. His stooped, low, 'C' posture on the bike would have loaded all his bodyweight through the stack of cotton reels (and none through the facets) and caused a greater than usual pressure on the low lumbar discs, without dissipating any force through the segments-squelching-forward effect of a natural lumbar lordosis. The vibration of the bike would have also compressed the discs faster.

To help get some lumbar hollow, I asked Graham to lie on his tummy, resting on his elbows in the Sphinx position, and while there, I helped his back settle into a deeper hollow by rotating his pelvis lightly from side to side. His back relaxed down more quickly than I might have expected, except for the L5–S1 segment which remained blocked. I decided to use the heel of my left foot to mobilise L5 because of its hard, brittle feel. By taking weight through my right foot on the sacrum and then alternately transferring my weight between the two, I started to loosen the bottom link of the spine. Graham found this a very comforting feeling. He enjoyed the sensation of the spine being prised apart as the sacrum was tipped back while pressure was kept on the L5 spinous process.

WARNING: Do not do this mobilisation at home.
Allow only a qualified professional to undertake this treatment.

I then showed him the squatting exercises (which open the back of the spine) which he was to repeat throughout the day, whenever he felt the low back tightening up. This also gave him the feeling of the segments being pulled apart and I suggested he might use the Pose of the Child exercise beforehand if his back felt too stiff to go straight into a squat.

Finally, I took Graham through the BackBlock routine, to be done daily, after the Sphinx and before the squatting. (Doing them in this order made sure that any unwanted facet jamming from the Sphinx was relieved by the BackBlock.)

Third treatment

Several weeks after Graham first started treatment he was far from better but signs of progress were evident. Although he could still not sit for any length of time, he was relieved that the exercises were making his back feel less gripped. He could also get himself out of pain when it came on. He had taken to breaking up his exercises throughout the day; doing another batch of squatting, rocking the knees to the chest, Sphinx and spinal rolling whenever he felt the back starting to stiffen. However, he still had moments of despair and wondered whether he should have the disc removed surgically. By this time, I was using my heel on L5 whenever he came in to see me, but his visits were more for me to evaluate his progress and modify his home routine.

Although his back still had its cobbled-from-within appearance he could bend much further forward. But the obvious rotating swivel had become much more marked, and his pelvis seemed to sit twisted on his legs. The swivel did not cause pain as he bent forward, (although he could feel it happening), but he noticed the twisted pelvis was worse when he was going through a more painful spate.

At this stage, I felt Graham was suffering more from the instability of the segment than simple disc prolapse. I also knew the pressure on the disc could not be relieved while the muscles in the back were causing it to work in this way. If we were not careful, the stiffness punctuated by the tiny slippage of L5 would re-inflame the restraining structures and increase the pressure on the nerve. It therefore became imperative to start tightening up the small intrinsic muscles across the L5–S1 interspace.

We started intrinsics exercises off the end of a table and quite quickly Graham was doing thirty at a stretch. He said his back felt good after these; it felt stronger and more able to put itself about. At the same time, we progressed to using the BackBlock on its end in the hope of pulling more fluid into the flaccid disc to make it more tense. Incorporated in the Block routine, Graham was now doing up to 400 curl ups per day, though not all at the one time. However, because of the potential ill-effects of the upper abdominal muscles shortening and causing the upper body to stoop forward, it was also important to start using the BackBlock under the upper back to avert this.

Although Graham had been using the BackBlock earlier—to move his centre of gravity back and establish a better alignment of his spine over its base—he needed to progress to using it on its middle edge (lengthwise and level with the top of the shoulders). He could stretch his pectoral muscles by sweeping his straight arms in broad semi-circles from the hips to above his head. Lengthening these muscles stops the shoulders being tethered forward, and makes it possible to thrust the chest out.

Fourth treatment

By the time I saw Graham ten months later, his spine looked 25 years younger. He was now using a kneeling chair to sit on at work (having spent between three and four months on the floor), but whenever he had to sit in a strange chair he would stiffen again. As a final progression of the intrinsics strengthening exercises, I asked him to do vigorous toe touches and diagonal toes touches with the feet spread wide. Not only did the energetic bending suck the segments apart and encourage a better fluid exchange through the lower discs, it also demanded a higher level of coordination between the tummy and the two groups of back muscles. His back felt looser afterwards.

He often got up and touched his toes after sitting at his desk but he would need to squat first to get the spine pulled out; then it would bend more easily without a tendency to give way. All other parts of the treatment regimen remained in place. In total, he was doing 30–40 minutes of exercise, though it was broken up through the day.

Fifth treatment

Two years later, Graham's back was much better though still not 100 per cent. It took over eighteen months before he could use a normal office chair but he was able to go running again (once every ten days) and not suffer ill effects. He had found yoga was a great benefit for the variety of different freedoms it created, and had included a couple of the twisting postures in his schedule.

Whenever he felt the stiffness mounting, he would mobilise L5 in the Sphinx position which always gave him more freedom to go on with. If he wanted to resume cycling, I asked him to use the sit-up-and-beg posture of the smaller bikes or the flat-out posture of the racing cyclists with the forearm support handle bars. Either way, the central core of his spine would not take the brunt of the pressure.

6 Segmental instability

This is the end condition in the breakdown of a segment when it becomes potentially loose, like a weak link in a chain.

WHAT IS SEGMENTAL INSTABILITY?

Segmental instability is the opposite to segmental stiffness; it is caused when one link in the spine is too loose instead of too stiff. It happens when the two main stabilising structures of a segment—both the disc and the facet joints—become stretched and weakened by a degenerative process. Full-blown segmental instability is extremely rare and may be incurable by conservative means because so many systems are in trouble at once—all fuelling one another—and the sources of pain may be multiple.

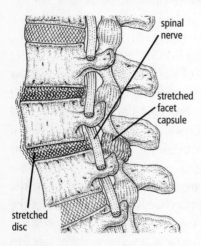

Figure 6.1 When the fibrous union of both disc and facets becomes stretched, the segment must rely on the primitive bony notching of the facets to keep itself in place.

However, there is another kind of 'muscular' instability of the spine, brought on by a short-lived underactivity of the deeper muscles of the spine, because a spinal segment is inflamed. This fleeting lapse can expose frank instability when muscle power deserts a structurally weakened segment. Conversely, symptoms of 'real' instability can be kept under control as long as the deep-acting muscles do their best to keep the segment stable. This shows how imperative it is to get the spine working properly once it has developed bad movement patterns from pain. But it also shows the scope of intrinsic exercises in keeping instability problems at bay.

'Real' instability develops when primary weakness of the disc eventually translates across to the facets, or when primary laxity of the facets translates across to the disc. Both structures share almost evenly the job of gluing the spinal segments together and holding them secure when the spine moves. If one of them fails, a greater load is transmitted to the other. As soon as the segment is loose in both front *and* back compartments, it can jostle around in the column with only the primitive bony notching mechanism of the facets and the power of the intrinsic muscles keeping it intact.

The confusing thing about instability is that it is often hard to pick up. The defenses of the spine can be so strong your back can simply feel super-stiff. It is impossible to sense any segmental looseness because the spinal segments are all jammed together as one block. The weak link may only come to light when the spasm starts to ease and the spine goes to bend. As the spine goes over without being properly braced, the loose vertebra slips forward like a drawer slipping out of a chest of drawers as it tips over.

There are other circumstances where a loose vertebra moves, in a much more low-grade way, every time the spine bends. This may not be especially worrying; you sense a tiny click or slip in your lower back as you go over, or a small wriggle in the movement, which you cannot prevent happening. In other circumstances, there may be a small arc of pain, just after your spine leaves the vertical, whereafter it moves freely and you go right to your toes. Returning to upright, there is a similar catch of pain just as you near the top. This is exactly the point where the segment slips.

Sometimes your spine continues on for months with the segment slipping this way every time you bend. There is always a degree of background stiffness but if you do something to hurt your back, it will start getting stiffer. The stiffer the muscles become, the more awkwardly your back moves and the louder the clicks get—until the stiffness becomes so limiting there is very little movement at all, and the clicking stops. At this point, depending on other circumstances (such as how tired you are; whether you are unwell) the defenses of the spine can reveal themselves as not up to the job of protecting the weak link. If an action is awkward as well as weighty, or if there is a mishap while lifting, you will have an ominous sense of your spine starting to give way. Before you can stop it, you are caught and your whole back collapses, doubled over like a broken reed.

Although the degree of uncontrolled movement of the vertebra is minuscule, it still constitutes 'unstable' activity. The micro-trauma from the repetitive slippage and the giving-way incidents all add up to inflame the structures trying to hold everything in place.

The most worrying movement is the forward gliding one (segmental shear), because the spine has fewer restraints to control it. Excessive forward tipping is not so bad, except that this facilitates shear. By tipping too much the vertebra disengages the facet lock and is free to slide forward more. This has the potential to slice transversely through the soft spinal cord, like a meat-slicer through a sausage.

When the loose vertebra goes to slip there can be a feeling of the weak link about to give way. This usually happens when the spine moves forward from the vertical position, like a stack of children's building blocks coming undone as soon as it leaves the stability of being upright. It can also happen when the spine is stretched across in the slung-out position, such as when leaning across to make a bed.

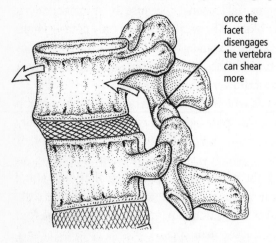

once the facet disengages the vertebra can shear more

As much as anything, it is the guarding reaction of the tummy and spinal muscles which brings you down. They all clench automatically which takes your breath away, but unlike the out-of-the-blue facet locking episode described in Chapter 4, you have a sense of the familiar; you can feel danger coming and you can stop it before it reaches the critical point. The muscles growlingly go on guard, flickering in a menacing sort of way as you go to do something awkward; a warning sign to stop the movement and backtrack out of it before it goes too far.

Figure 6.2 We have few restraints to control the vertebra shearing—we can only do so by controlling tip. Thus, with an unstable segment, you must always bend with a tight tummy and rounded back.

If you go on for a while without the back folding up under pressure, the incremental slippage can stop happening. One day you realise the stiffness has gone, and the clicking beneath the surface has also faded. Your back moves better as the harmony of the muscles returns. This usually happens with a fitness or weight control binge, particularly if it involves tummy strengthening as well. It means the weak link has made itself more secure by becoming stiffer, or the segmental muscles across the link have taken to working better. This precarious truce is more or less maintainable (unless you do heavy pushing work), but the former rumblings cannot be wholly ignored. The weak link will always be the first to give way when your back is next put to the test.

When the weak link is stressed, pain may not come on immediately; returning stiffness may be the first clue. This gets more and more noticeable a few days after chopping down a tree, or taking a car trip over a rough road, and then a gnawing pain starts in the leg. The weak link is more susceptible to knocks and bangs passing through the spine, and slowly the level of inflammation rises as the segment is squeezed by the tightening muscles.

Diagnosis

Diagnosing full-blown instability can be difficult because of the complexity of the pain picture. There can be so much pain, it is hard to know where to start. Action X-rays rarely show the segment opening and closing more than it should do because the spinal defenses are much too clever for that. The surrounding muscles splint the loose vertebra and make it appear stiff. A discogram can show internal degradation of the disc, but the most definitive sign of instability is none of these: it is the presence of tooth-like extensions of bone around both the interbody and facet joints.

With longstanding instability, the disc-vertebra complex develops small outgrowths of bone around the perimeter of the disc, where it meets the vertebral body. These are thought to serve two purposes: first to provide a broader base of bone for the disc wall taking a greater load and second, to support the spine's valiant attempt to stiffen the loose link. Here the spurs act as reinforcement for the fibres of the disc wall to tie themselves down to the bone and provide stronger anchorage for the stretching wall.

Similar changes occur in the facet joints when the primary instability is there. The lower facet surface remoulds itself to make a more enveloping lip of bone which curls up around the upper facet surface to hold it in place. In the trade, these are called 'wrap around bumpers' and they too are thought to be an ingenious attempt by the body to make the joint more secure. The bony cupping traps the upper vertebra and reduces its ability to slide out of joint.

However, these bony outgrowths around the end-plate of the disc and/or the facet joint only come about when a vertebra has been wobbling about for a long time—by which time it is virtually incurable through spinal strengthening exercises. And it is for this reason that 'weakness' instabilities, when they occur, must receive our full attention.

A great deal of focus must be given to re-educating proper free-flowing spinal movement when the back is bad—in case some freak movement creeps in under the spine's guard and wrenches the unprotected problem link. This will create an unstable segment where there was none before. In fact, that is the central aim of this book: to prevent a stiff spinal link becoming an unstable one, or better still to prevent a stiff link developing in the first place.

Not uncommonly, the segment soldiers on valiantly with its chronically

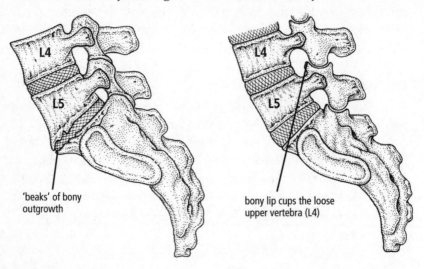

'beaks' of bony
outgrowth

bony lip cups the loose
upper vertebra (L4)

Figure 6.3 'Saw-toothed' projections where the disc joins the vertebra are a sure sign the front compartment is loose.

Figure 6.4 'Wrap-around bumpers' develop where the lower facet surfaces remould an enveloping lip to contain the upper surfaces.

stretched ligaments, coping quite well with the anomalous movement of both front and back compartments. Often, it is when you do something extra to hurt the back that things flare up; the facet swells more or the bulging disc starts impinging on the nearby nerve root. Savage, intolerable leg pain often brings things to a head—and often to the point of the surgeon's knife.

Spinal surgery

Operating on spinal instability involves surgically joining the loose upper vertebra to the lower one by inserting two large titanium screws through both facet joints and then packing out the evacuated disc space with bone chips taken from the pelvic bone. This is called a spinal fusion. It is usually done after first removing the flaccid disc (and sometimes part of the facet joint) in order to relieve the pressure on the spinal nerve root. These procedures are called discectomy and partial facetectomy.

As you might imagine, careful operative technique is of the essence with spinal surgery because prolific scar formation causes so many more problems. If the scarring becomes invasive, it can be just as space-occupying and obtrusive as the structure deemed worthy of removal in the first place. In particular, the nerve root can be slowly strangled by the growth of adhesions, eventually causing the same symptoms of pressure on the nerve, and the old pain starts up again. Postoperative adhesions are similar to the post-inflammatory condition called 'root sleeve fibrosis' described with facet arthropathy and chronic disc prolapse (see Chapters 3 and 5).

The other complication of spinal fusion is the strain translated to the next working level up (L4 if L5 has been fused, or L3 if L4 and L5 have been fused). Both are almost flimsy compared to the robust L5–S1 junction and are ill-equipped to act as the seat of spinal movement. They are not bedded deeply in the pelvis like L5, nor do they have the august ilio-lumbar ligament to lash them down. Thus they are progressively over-taxed by routine movement. The problem usually takes several years to manifest and affects L3 more seriously than L4. Intrinsic spinal strengthening is therefore a critical part of a post-fusion regimen.

CAUSES OF SEGMENTAL INSTABILITY

- Primary breakdown of the disc
- Primary breakdown of the facet joints
- Incompetence of the 'bony catch' mechanism of the facet joints
- Weakness and poor coordination of the trunk muscles

Primary breakdown of the disc

In the later stages of breakdown of a stiff spinal segment the nucleus degrades to such a degree that the disc becomes like an inert flattened washer. It is so lacking in internal pressure, it can no longer prime itself and spring-load its vertebra to keep the segment taut as the spine bends forward.

Over time, the passive non-performance of the disc means the vertebra simply shears forward as the spine bends, tugging and stretching the disc as it goes. Like a perishing car tyre veering onto its wall as it rounds a corner, the flaccid disc is gradually destroyed by its own vertebra's runaway movement.

When the disc has no stuffing, the constant weight of the spine bearing down through the weak link is further cause for breakdown. With its much reduced intra-discal pressure, the disc cannot fight back and the main brunt of the load is borne by the walls. They have nowhere to go but billow outwards, like a cardboard box crumpling when a weight is put on top.

With long periods of sitting the distension of the walls becomes more marked because of the fluid loss. As the upper vertebra settles closer to the lower one, the disc bulges around its circumference like an inflatable rubber collar, and the two vertebrae almost touch. The back may slew sideways on the sick disc to lift the pouting wall off the nearby spinal nerve; it may remain kinked into a windswept 'S' bend after rising from sitting, and take time to disappear. A sciatic scoliosis like this is often more pronounced after attending a seminar for a few days or after a busy period of sitting writing reports.

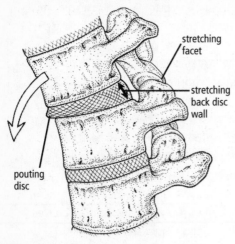

Figure 6.5 The lack of pressure in a sick disc means the spine skids and slews forward on it whenever you bend.

This process of breakdown can be greatly speeded up by a percussive injury through the length of the spine if the nucleus has already degenerated and is looking for a way out. The impact can blow a vent through the thin cartilage of the vertebral end-plate and squirt the degraded nuclear material into the blood-saturated honeycomb bone (spongiosa) in the vertebra above or below. End-plate fracture when the disc is healthy will not result in the nucleus breaking out, although it may cause rapid deterioration of the disc's health.

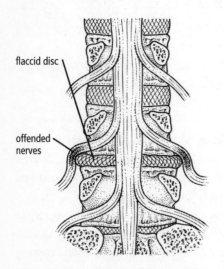

Figure 6.6 With the disc bulging all around like an inflatable rubber collar, the nerves on both sides are vulnerable.

Once the nuclear material has penetrated the bone, the blood cells in the spongiosa attack the toxic disc material as an unwelcome foreign substance, and an auto-immune reaction sets up. This does not limit itself to the dislodged material but continues back through the communicating hole into what is left of the disc. The remnant disc is then devoured by the auto-immune reaction, leaving a flaccid fibrous bag of scar tissue where the main bulk of the disc once was. This process is called *primary disc disease*.

Not surprisingly, this is a back problem common in the armed forces. Soldiers who train over assault courses are particularly susceptible through landing heavily on both feet. Parachutists are also at risk, as are pilots who use ejection seats: they all suffer similar traumatic shocks up through the spine which may be painless at the time. It is also the complaint of the weekend gardener. Forceful tugging at a stubborn root, or unaccustomed heavy lifting, can punch a hole though the cartilaginous end-plate which is insufficiently 'seasoned' to tolerate the force.

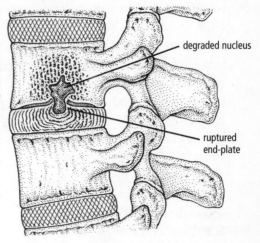

Figure 6.7 Disc breakdown can escalate when impact up through the spine squidges a semi-degraded nucleus into the neighbouring vertebra.

Once the disc has become incompetent, the segment will remain stable in the column only as long as the other main control mechanism of the facets is up to the task. Depending on the stresses on the facets, the strain will eventually be felt there and the facet capsules are the first to complain.

Primary breakdown of the facet joints

Segmental instability can also start off when facet joints develop severe arthritic change (see Chapter 3). With poor joint lubrication and the friction of the joint surfaces chafing, the cartilage buffer within the joint is worn down, making the two opposing bones ride closer together. This causes the joint capsule to pucker and the joint develops excessive play during activity—even though in time it ingeniously moulds its lower bone surface into a cup-shape to cope. Even so, the joint slips around with movement and articular destruction picks up apace.

Sometimes, instability can spread from repeated facet locking episodes (see Chapter 4). With each mini-dislocation, the capsule is traumatised and healthy tissue is replaced by scar tissue. As the capsule becomes weaker it also loses elastic recoil, thus making it harder to keep its joint snugly together.

However, facet locking typically affects one facet only, so instability is less likely to spread across the whole segment from this problem.

Incompetence of the 'bony catch' mechanism of the facet joints

You can also develop segmental instability when the solid bone-to-bone backup of the facet joints becomes incompetent. This can happen in three ways: a congenital malformation (called spina bifida) where the facet joints fail to develop properly in utero; a physical break in the bony neck at the bottom of the catch mechanism, usually caused by trauma (called spondylolisthesis); when the bony neck of the catch mechanism gradually elongates, like toffee stretching (called spondylolysis).

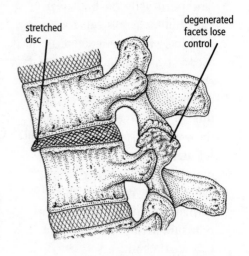

Figure 6.8 Facet breakdown, which leaves the articular cartilage eroded and the capsules slack, can throw great strain on the disc.

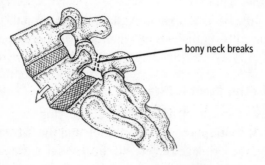

bony neck breaks

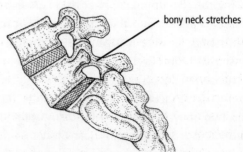

bony neck stretches

Figure 6.9 With spondylolisthesis, a break in the neck of bone below the lower facet surface can make the locking mechanism incompetent, so the vertebra slips forward. With spondylolysis, the bone 'stretches' rather than breaks.

In all cases, the bony catch of the facet's locking mechanism fails to prevent the upper vertebra slipping forward on the lower one. Without the lock of bone against bone—like a row of fingers of one hand hooked up against the fingers of the other—both the disc and facet capsules slowly stretch, letting the upper vertebra gradually slip over the abyss.

As dramatic as a spondylolisthesis can look on X-ray, with an overhang of sometimes as much as half the upper vertebra, it can be quite stable. The flattening of the disc as the vertebra pulls forward causes the disc wall to harden as it bunches down. Barring some fluke additional mishap knocking it loose (like a hard fall on the bottom or a scrum collapsing in a rugby game) the segment may remain symptom-free for years.

I see this in clinical practice all the time: people with a low-grade backache unwittingly harbouring a fairly advanced slip, to have it flare up only when they suffer some minor mishap. The new trauma may cause an additional slip of a millimetre or two but even so, the upper vertebra usually settles down securely on the lower one quite quickly. The lesser symptoms of a stiff segment then return.

It is not unusual to break the neck of a facet with impact through an over-arched lower back, and we see this often enough with fast bowlers landing heavily on their leading leg at cricket. You can also break the catch mechanism with a fall on your bottom, and an astonishing number of the Inuit population have spondylolisthesis from falls on ice. Some of these cases remain chronically unstable, with fractures on both sides of the bony ring failing to unite. The back then permanently harbours a low-grade ache and a tendency to give way when caught off guard or with an awkward move-ment. Broken bones and all, it is often surprising how little pain there is.

Weakness and poor coordination of the trunk muscles

When an intervertebral disc dries and flattens due to the degenerative process, the intrinsic muscles which work the upper vertebra have a harder job. Their angle of pull is reduced which means their already poor mechanical advantage is reduced further. Thus it is harder for muscular control of the segment to compensate for weakness of the other two stabilisers, and the vertebra is more vulnerable to slip.

Full-blown instability can also develop from fleeting 'weakness' of a segment because the back is suffering pain; a temporary alteration in muscle balance can cause the segment to loosen more quickly. This happens for two reasons: one volitional (conscious) and the other automatic.

The *volitional element* is because of the way you use your back when it hurts—avoiding bending and making your knees do all the work. People usually do this because they think they are doing the right thing. They feel that bending their knees and keeping their back straight will make things better. Over the years this has been reinforced by old-fashioned back care programs, in the belief it put less pressure on the discs. We now know this to be wrong, and furthermore, that using the back this way only makes matters worse.

It emphasises the use of the stronger, clumsier muscles of the spine while under-utilising the smaller, fine-acting ones which control the individual segments. Thus the spine operates en masse in a bulky, non-bending fashion, and loses subtle undulating motion throughout its length. This makes it feel precarious in complex postures and safe only when it does simple actions like a robot. As it gets stiffer and weaker, it becomes increasingly vulnerable to shearing strains at one of its lower links.

Even preliminary efforts to make the spine bend properly at this stage will improve things—and despite your wariness, you often find it happens quite easily. After two or three times touching your toes (preferably with the knees bent like a gorilla so tight hamstrings do not restrict you), your back immediately feels freer and more supple.

The *automatic element* of muscle dysfunction is a little more complicated and is more likely to happen if there is inflammation in the back. If there is an irritable disc or facet joint, the finer-acting deep muscles can be 'paralysed' by the dominant activity of the long back muscles, even though their main purpose is protective. But the finer group can also inhibit as a pre-emptive measure, to spare the inflamed segment excessive compression of the muscle working normally.

Some speculation

It is possible, though not documented, that transversus abdominus, the deepest acting tummy muscle, reduces activity if there is primary inflammation of the interbody joint—that is, a stiff spinal segment—because its action clenches the cotton reels together vertically. Lighter neurocentral compression may lessen the pain, even though it ultimately hastens instability.

On the other hand, multifidus may automatically dampen its activity if there is inflammation of the facet joints. Although this spares the irritable facet from compression, it inevitably results in poorer control of the vertebra's tail and makes it more vulnerable to shear and rotational instability.

Whether first up there is over-activity of the dominant group or automatic inhibition of the deeper ones, there is no doubt that one end fuels the other.

The stronger group gets stronger and the weaker one gets weaker.

This is the way it works: whenever there is pain in the back, the long back muscles develop 'protective reflex spasm' which splints everything straight and limits movement. They lock up the length of the spine, like guy-ropes holding a flagpole in a gale, jamming its base into the ground and making it bow in the middle under the strain. As the low back compresses more, the intrinsic muscles relinquish their hold. This leaves all the spinal segments— but particularly a problem one at the base—more likely to shear forward when the spine bends.

The mechanism also works in reverse. Once the unstable segment reveals a tendency to shear, a vicious cycle sets in. As if sensing the weak link, the long muscles clench the spine even more. This makes the whole back board-like, but further disables the control of the segments. Then a self-fuelling cycle gears up. The spine develops a brittle veneer of stiffness which makes it awkward to move, and the weak link inside is ever more prone to shear.

Patients often half recognise this themselves. Their back becomes increasingly sore, with stiffness extending right up to the neck. It also keeps giving way at the base if they don't protect it. They lose confidence with anything involving bending, fearing they might end up in a heap on the floor, and they become hidebound by a multitude of constraints. They creep about, taking the path of least resistance and planning every move, even down to picking up a teacup.

THE WAY THIS BACK BEHAVES
The acute phase

Acute segmental instability is arrived at after being chronic for some years and suddenly taking a turn for the worse. Being unfit, putting on weight and sleeping in a very soft bed are background factors which together can tip the balance, but strong physical exertion is often the final straw. Strenuous pushing activities, such as pushing a car, are often linked to the back getting worse, no doubt from the backward shearing action of the spine on the flaccid disc which it is ill-equipped to prevent.

Then the variety of symptoms—and the emergence of new ones—can make the problem very difficult to unravel. Except for extra rigidity in the back, its worst features are often indistinguishable from acute disc prolapse, with an angry pain and paraesthesia (disturbed sensation) down the leg. What differentiates instability is the long history leading up to the present crisis.

At the peak of the acute phase, the long back muscles stand up like cables, making it impossible to hump your low back and bend. Try as you might, the muscles will not let go. Everything appears stuck, like a puppet with its strings pulled too tight, and then you develop a crippling pain down the leg when finally the nerve is affected by so much inflammation in the local area. At this point, the back will be doubly disinclined to bend: both to ward off any slippage at the weak link and to avoid stretching the inflamed nerve.

You will be uncomfortable in most positions, even turning over in bed, because your spine has lost its serpentine control of all the segments as it undulates across the mattress. You will know from experience the best way to do this is either rolling over like a log, or very slowly with the tummy braced, so the spine does not disjoint at the weak link. But if the instability is severe and the leg pain intractable, you will hardly know what to do with yourself. You will be pathetically crippled by your leg, and only comfortable lying in the foetal position with a pillow between your knees. Sitting may be impossible and walking may be reduced to a shuffle by the nerve root's painful inability to take stretch (see Chapter 5). Invariably at this point the condition needs surgical intervention.

What causes the acute pain?

With acute instability, there will be intense backpain, quite probably from more than one structure at once. It is arguable whether more pain will come from the side of the motion segment which became unstable first, although the facets—with their propensity for inflammatory response and their sophisticated nerve supply—will always register a lot more pain than a disc. Broadly speaking, the true picture of instability is often a time-lapsed composite of the different conditions which have afflicted the segment during its long course of breakdown.

At one and the same time there may be symptoms from the stretched disc wall (see Chapter 2), from a localised bulge in the wall (see Chapter 5) and from the inflamed facet joint (see Chapter 3). As a result, there may be central back pain in addition to a one-sided back pain. There may also be sciatica and numbness and weakness in the leg from both the capsular inflammation and the disc prolapse. And just to complicate matters, there may also be referred pain in the leg from the facet joint problem. It certainly is complicated.

The sub-acute phase

If there is no pain down the leg, it is still possible to recover from this problem without surgery. If you persevere, your back will grudgingly regain segmental strength and learn to bend, especially if you pull your tummy in and hump the low back first. Soon enough you will notice a tell-tale wriggle or kinking movement in the lower back emerging through the stiffness, even when your back is still quite cast.

The wriggle may come about as your spine tries to avoid skidding on the flaccid disc. Watching the movement happening from behind, the spine appears to do a lateral semi-circular movement as if attempting to roll around the rim of the flattened disc as it goes forward. It can go around either the left or right side of the rim but either way, the aberrant movement appears to be more unnerving than painful. Until you build up the strength of your intrinsics, you can minimise this by pulling your tummy in hard, both before you bend over and nearly at the top on the way up again.

With the widespread armour-plating of the muscles you often feel more pain in your upper back as stiffness spreads to the better-off regions. Sometimes there is soreness right up between your shoulder blades and you may have headaches as well. Sufferers often seek spinal manipulation at this point, which is ill-advised. Although manipulation comes into its own with other spinal conditions—particularly segmental stiffness if the vertebra is twisted on its axis, or with facet joint locking—there is no way, for even the most experienced operators, to accurately localise the manipulative thrust to the stiff segments while sparing the weak one.

The so-called 'million dollar roll' (where the patient is put on his or her side and the low back clicked one way then the other) often wrenches the weak link, even though the sense of release which coincides with the characteristic popping sound can be profound. However, people usually get increasingly uneasy about having the same treatment over and over again when there is no long-term improvement. With manipulations getting more frequent, and the benefit shorter-lived, many decide to look deeper and search out a more permanent (if not instantaneous) solution—and to understand what was wrong in the first place.

You are usually at your most comfortable sitting, because the reduced hollowing in the low back lessens the forward inclination of the lumbar vertebrae and thus the tendency for the weak one to slip forward. But rising from sitting to standing can be agony. There is often a painful catch as you straighten and you may have to push yourself up through the final part with your hands on your thighs. Basically you will be unhappy about feeling the movement of the vertebra, and there is good reason for this. You will always be on guard against it letting you down.

You will know from experience that the more clicking and grating there is in your back, the stiffer it will become. As the back tightens, there is a dawning of the familiar pain down your leg, which starts off as an ache and then turns into a cramp. Sometimes the leg pain arrives before your back stiffens but either way, the re-emergence of familiar symptoms is a sign the link is inflaming again. It usually corresponds with a period of excess, when your exercise routine has lapsed or you have put on a few extra pounds.

Then you find it increasingly awkward to do everyday things. You may notice your actions becoming more laboured before the pain becomes obvious. Even something as simple as picking a belt up from the chair can become a farce. Your back stays ramrod straight and you feel safer bending sideways with your bottom out and bending your knees, rather than going down normally.

The chronic phase

You can cope with a chronically unstable back indefinitely, if you can stop the weak link inflaming. You are usually the best judge of the way to do this, as you are more in tune with your back than most practitioners. Although pain may not be a big factor with the low grade instability, you are strikingly susceptible to minor misadventure. Strengthening of the weak link is imperative, to stop you being catapulted into difficulty at a moment's notice.

With chronic instability, there is muscle stiffness all over the back and a soreness which is pretty well localised to the problem level. However, the level of pain is unpredictable and varies with what the back has to endure. Something as simple as stepping off a curb can set it off—because the lack of support allows the spine to strain at the weak link—but so can heavy jarring exertions which rattle the link.

When the condition is truly quiescent, the back rarely gives way when you go to bend forward and you hardly ever feel it clicking and grinding. You can set off a peaceful back however (and you will be annoyed with yourself that you should have known better) by over-doing sustained bending activity, such as vacuum cleaning or laborious sweeping or raking, or pushing anything heavy, like a wardrobe. (It is always better to turn around and push with your back.)

Difficulty with straightening after bending is a sure sign things are wrong. Because the pooling of interstitial fluid causes a transient wedge of water-logging at the back of the over-mobile segment, it is difficult to close the gapping at the back of the spine to let you straighten. For the first few steps you get about like an old man with knees bent and bottom out, and both hands on the back of your hips to help winch you straight.

More often than not it amounts to nothing more than that. Your back feels normal again within a few steps and the stiffness fades. But occasionally you stay doubled over and a generalised stiffness sets in across the back which you cannot throw off. It can linger for several days, making it increasingly awkward to do things—until you do something thoughtlessly, your back gives way, and you are tipped into an acute phase again.

Although the mishap usually happens when your back is caught off guard, it is unlike acute facet locking (see Chapter 4) in that you can sense your back getting ready to slip at the weak link and you can avoid it by stopping the movement short. Sometimes if you are quick enough you can stop yourself collapsing to the floor by getting your hands to your thighs as your back gives way. Then you can unfurl yourself to vertical by thrusting your pelvis forward under the spine and pushing up with your hands.

You will see from the self treatment section how important it is to stop the spine stiffening up all over at this point; it is essential to prevent your back getting so rigid that the deep muscles lose control of the individual segments. As soon as possible you have to get down on the floor and roll back and forth along the spine to prevent the segments jamming up.

What causes the chronic pain?

The pain of chronic instability is probably a combination of the micro-trauma stretching the fibres of both the disc and the facets, and the compression of the runaway segment by the spine's defence mechanisms. In practice however, it is impossible to differentiate between the two.

As fibres right across the motion segment are progressively damaged by the excessive movement, toxins are released which stimulate free nerve endings, thus alerting the brain that all is not well. This manifests in the form of pain—both from the disc wall and the facets—plus a greater or lesser degree of muscle spasm. The spasm is not only painful in itself but contributes in its own way to more instability.

Meanwhile, there can also be pain from the vascular engorgement of the weak link when it is locked up tight by the large muscles of the spine holding the whole back stiff. When the cable-like muscles clench all the segments together, as if they were in a mechanical vice, the weak problem link in the middle can bloat up painfully because the circulation through it is hampered by the compression.

Then, you not only get pain from the oxygen deprivation (anoxia) of the tissues (because there is no fresh blood coming through to bring more oxygen), but you also get pain from the rising concentration of metabolites or waste products in the tissues because the old blood cannot get away.

WHAT YOU CAN DO ABOUT IT
The aims of self treatment for instability

The immediate aim when treating acute instability is to dampen the inflammation of the weak link so the nerve settles down. Initially, this involves relaxing the muscle spasm to let the pressure off the segment and allow a better circulation to pass through. Treatment in this phase is exactly the same as for the acute disc prolapse, with an emphasis on rocking the knees to the chest to open the back of the spine. It is then important to establish better movement patterns as soon as possible, so the spine does not keep skidding on the flaccid disc. Reverse curl-ups start to strengthen the tummy and help switch off the long back muscles.

As soon as the pain is on the move, it is important to start treating the back 'normally' so the intrinsic muscles play a more active role knitting the loose link together, and the natural ebb and flow of movement helps to pump the congestion away. Toe touching exercises should start as soon as possible so that the spine gets accustomed to bending with segmental control, and together with squatting and the BackBlock they help puff up the disc to make it more tense. Encouraging the flattened disc to imbibe fluid not only takes pressure off the walls but gives the intrinsic muscles a better angle of pull to stabilise the segment. However, toe touching works the back hard when it is still quite reactive, and it needs a lot of spinal rolling to break up the stiffness which comes on.

In the final stages of rehabilitation, the emphasis is on spinal strengthening so the weak link does not keep re-inflaming. This is done with horizontal intrinsic exercises off the end of a table. However, the muscular compression of the energetic unfurling action jams the segments together and can make the low back sore again. For this reason, the main intrinsic exercises should only be done three times a week, although it is necessary to continue toe touching, spinal rolling, rocking the knees and using the BackBlock, to disperse treatment soreness.

A typical treatment for acute instability

(See Chapter 7 for descriptions of all exercises and the correct way to do them.)

Purpose: Relieve muscle spasm, start the spine bending

Rocking knees to the chest (60 seconds)

Rest, knees crooked, feet flat on bed (30 seconds)

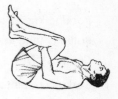

Rocking knees to the chest

Rest

Rocking knees to the chest

Reverse curl ups (five times)

Rest

Rocking knees to chest

Reverse curl ups

Rest

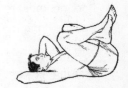

Rocking knees to the chest

Curl ups (five times)

Rest

Rocking knees to chest

Curl ups

Rest

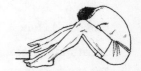

Rocking knees to the chest

Curl ups

Rest

Medication. Rest in bed. Repeat exercises every 30 minutes. If the curl ups cause pain in the leg, revert to reverse curl ups only.

A typical treatment for sub-acute instability

Purpose: Disperse inflammation from weak link, break up muscle spasm, re-establish segmental movement

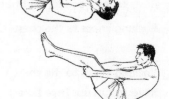

Rocking knees to the chest (60 seconds)
Rolling along the spine (15–30 seconds)
Curl ups (five times)

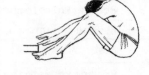

Rocking knees to the chest
Rolling along the spine
Curl ups

Rocking knees to the chest
Rolling along the spine
Curl ups

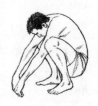

Rocking knees to the chest
Rolling along the spine
Curl ups

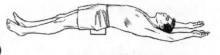

BackBlock (60 seconds)
Rocking knees to the chest (30 seconds)
Curl ups (15 times)

Squatting (30 seconds)
Toe touching (down and up three times)

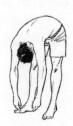

You may feel a click or a slipping movement in your back doing the curl ups. If this happens, suck your tummy in harder and do the exercise more slowly, attempting to hump your back as you go. If this fails, pull yourself up to a sitting position with the hands on the thighs and concentrate on the reverse journey to the floor. If the leg pain returns, revert to acute regimen for a couple of days.

A typical treatment for chronic instability

Purpose: Decompress spine to relieve pressure on the flaccid disc, strengthen the weak link, restore trunk coordination

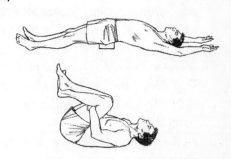

Rolling along the spine (15–30 seconds)

BackBlock (60 seconds)

Rocking knees to the chest (30 seconds)

Curl ups (15 times)

BackBlock

Rocking knees to the chest

Curl ups

Intrinsics (12–15 times)

Rocking knees to chest

Rolling along the spine

Curl ups (15 times)

Intrinsics

Rocking knees to chest

Rolling along the spine

Curl ups

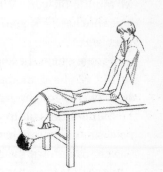

Repeat regimen three times a week indefinitely. Expect to feel tired and sore in the back after this strengthening program. If your back remains stiff for more than a couple of days afterwards, cut down to once a week only, for two to three weeks.

A CASE HISTORY OF SEGMENTAL INSTABILITY

Georgie is a 38-year-old ex-nurse who hurt her back in her mid-twenties catching a patient falling out of bed. At the time her problem was diagnosed as 'back strain'. She had a couple of days in bed and two weeks off work before resuming normal nursing duties.

She recovered quite well after the first episode but hurt her back again while nursing five years later. Georgie cannot recall much trouble from her back in the interim. The next mishap was when she was helping a radiographer pull an unconscious patient forward off an X-ray plate. The combination of a badly coordinated lift (the other girl let go too early, letting the patient loll over to the side) and the dead weight of the patient made her back go. She was standing side-on to the patient and although she had her legs in a wide step stance and her tummy braced, she felt a small click in the back. Soon after she felt slight lumbar discomfort but she also felt lightheaded and nauseated.

Next morning she woke up rigid, unable to move for the pain in her back. Over the next few days she developed a crippling pain down into the back thigh of the right leg. An X-ray revealed a Grade 1 (mild) spondylolisthesis at the L4–L5 level.

After this incident Georgie had no formal treatment except rest in bed and two months off work. When she returned to work she was given light clerical duties but her back continued to plague her until she gave up nursing several years later.

To some extent she kept her back under control herself by keeping fit and she did not have another flare-up for three years, when she went jogging after a twenty-four hour aeroplane flight. Her back seized during the run and she found it difficult to get herself home. She had a hot bath to relieve the increasing castness of her back but within a day she was immobile again with a severe pain down the back of the right leg to her calf.

By the time I saw her, she was very stiff and very sore; unable to bend and cautious about every move she made. During our first consultation she had one of those episodes every therapist dreads: before I had finished my examination, her back seized again when she was getting up from the prone position.

I assume that the simple probing of my hands exploring in her back had lessened the hold of the long spinal muscles enough to leave her vulnerable at the weak link as she went to lift up. Obviously their relaxation was not matched by the ability of her tummy or her deep spinal muscles to hold the link and it had slipped slightly as she changed her position.

Unwelcome as the seizing episode was at the time, it was ultimately good for Georgie to see how to handle the problem in the happening. As well as having me there with each step, she could see the time frames and the sort of repetition involved to bring about results. Even though she was frightened, as she had been facing similar circumstances in the past, this made-to-measure episode gave her the experience and confidence to weather similar mishaps in the future (if there were any!).

First treatment

Supporting the back of her head, I helped Georgie onto her back on the treatment couch. I then asked her to take one knee to her chest, and while she held it there with one hand, I helped her bring the other one up. With both knees between her interlaced fingers, I assisted her to gently bounce her knees to her chest.

After continuing for several minutes she was allowed to rest, by pulling her tummy in first and taking one foot down to the bed, then the other, so both feet were flat on the bed, knees crooked. After a short breather we resumed: first one leg to the chest, then the other, then rocking both gently so her bottom began to lift off the bed as the back of her spine began to round and the segments gap open.

This was repeated for fifteen to twenty minutes. After each repeat, she could place her feet back on the bed more easily, without her back going into protective spasm. Apart from loosening the spine by unjamming the spinal segments, the rocking routine was preparation for the curl up exercise which we needed to start as soon as possible.

Georgie was relatively comfortable on her back, holding both knees, although she was wary of pushing the movement too far and tugging the weak link in her back. This possibility lessened as she relaxed and chatted more animatedly. Eventually she noticed that her legs came up more freely and her bottom lifted off the bed further. She could also rock her knees through a wider range of movement without her low back feeling as if it would grab, in guarding mode, to steady the movement.

When starting the curl ups Georgie's apprehension about hurting her back was almost more of a problem than doing it. I helped her up by holding both hands, although after the first two or three, her former fitness showed through. She started doing them quite well herself, by using her tummy to make a proper curling action, rather than her hip muscles bringing her up in a dangerous slewing off-centre action with the back straight.

In several repeat sessions we did as many curl ups as she could at one time. I watched the quality of the movement to see she didn't jar the back or veer off-centre as fatigue crept in.

As Georgie dressed to go home, she was already nearly through the setback which could have laid her up for weeks. However, she still felt her tummy could not hold her up and I noticed that she bent down cautiously, bending her knees to pick up her clothes from the chair. She also walked slowly without swinging her hips but she was straight and her spine was in good alignment.

She had instructions to get down onto the floor as soon as she got home, to loosen her back again, because it would tighten up on the way home. This was to be followed with more curl ups (up to 15 at a time) and then she was to go to bed for the remainder of the day. The knee rocking and curl ups were to be repeated before going to sleep that night, and the same again on waking (bearing in mind the back would be a lot stiffer in the morning). I did not suggest she have a muscle relaxant or anti-inflammatory drugs to speed up recovery but if her back had taken longer to relax after the seizing episode, I would have.

Second treatment

Georgie arrived the next day for treatment feeling much as she had after the previous day; still wary that her back would let her down, but without marked muscle spasm to limit her movement.

The treatment proceeded faster. It was quicker getting her down on her back and less nerve-racking getting the knees up and locked on her chest. Her legs hinged more easily and her bottom immediately came up a distance from the couch. In short, the back felt lighter and more spontaneous and the curl ups were freer and took less effort.

By this time, I felt it safe to ask Georgie to lie on her tummy again, face down over a pillow, so I could feel what was going on in her back. I kept away from the spondylolisthesis (L4–5) and manually tested the other spinal segments. The lumbo-sacral level was particularly immobile with old thickening and recent puffy swelling (oedema) around the facet joint on the right. It was interesting that deep pressure here (with the elbow) reproduced some of her familiar right thigh pain.

This pain indicated that the unstable segment above was not solely responsible for her leg symptoms. It showed that the stiffness of the L5 segment was still a major source of pain, and furthermore the presence of the instability problem would have increased the protective muscle spasm, thus intensifying the symptoms from this stiffer level. In practice this is a common enough finding; the unstable level sends out less pain than neighbouring stiffer ones.

I mobilised the stiff L5 segment manually with quite sturdy forward gliding techniques, and followed up with similar loosening techniques of the right facet joint. Then, for the purposes of future self treatment, I emphasised the importance of spinal rolling to loosen the chronic jamming of the bottom segment. This was done by attempting to pivot on L5, with the knees quite un-bent so that the leg leverage was long enough to balance her over the lumbo-sacral area. Although this is quite strenuous for the tummy muscles, Georgie was able to balance there and feel the gradual softening of the muscles as they let the spine down into a rocker shape. After pivoting for a minute or so each time she relaxed to the floor for a breather and then repeated it another two times.

Not only did this ease the pain coming from the stiff link, but more importantly, it freed up L5 to contribute more movement, thus taking the onus off the over-mobile L4. An unstable link is always much happier once its neighbours are made more mobile. The spine immediately starts to move better as normality creeps in.

Mobilising L5 by rolling along the spine was followed by more rocking the knees to the chest, interspersed with 15 curl ups each time, up to 45 in total. Both spinal rolling and rocking the knees to the chest were to be continued at home at two hourly intervals throughout each day until the next treatment five days later. She no longer had to remain in bed, although it was suggested she might lie down briefly in the afternoon if her back was getting tired and stiff.

Third treatment

By this time, Georgie was already nearly painfree. The first part of this treatment consisted of more manual loosening of the stiff segments above and below the loose L4, followed by more curl ups, done faster and for longer. Then the physical elongation of the spine was started. This firstly meant squats which pull the spinal segments apart at the base, and then toe-touching which stretches the long back muscles while strengthening the deeper intrinsic muscles.

The squats are an important first measure because they make it so much easier for the spine to bend. Holding onto a firm ledge, Georgie went right down, with her bottom almost touching the floor. She felt a marked pulling sensation in the lower back which she could intensify both by widening her knees (keeping the feet together) and sucking her tummy in hard. Bouncing gently in this position she could feel the spine elongating cog by cog. As she rose, she used the power of her thighs, and pulled her tummy in hard to spear herself up straight.

Bending forward for the toe touches the first time was not easy. An in-built wariness that her spine might fold up made it difficult to get past first base. To make it easier, I suggested she bend her knees and use her hands to climb down her thighs. Once down, she could hang there for a few seconds with her hands almost touching the floor, stretching her spine, even though her hamstrings did not stretch.

I stressed the importance of humping her low back to keep it round as she bent forward. This she did by tightening her bottom and sucking the tummy in hard against the spine. As always, it is imperative to bend the spine forward 'around' the pocket of high intra-abdominal pressure which keeps the segments braced. Going forward in the wrong way, by bending at the hips with the belly relaxed, allows the spine to concave which takes the tension off the ligaments and lets the segments shear forward as the spine goes over. This would produce a nasty jab of pain and make the back fold up.

The return journey back to upright required nearly as much care as going down. Attention was needed to make an unfurling action from bent over position to upright. From the base up, the spine needed to be straightened, each segment slotting back in place on the vertebra below with a similar humping action to maintain tension. The direct action of both transversus abdominus and multifidus kept the runaway segment clenched in place in the column and pulled its tail down. It unfurled all the segments, in a wave-like motion up through the spine, the head coming up last.

Georgie was surprised how quickly she got the knack of bending and straightening in this controlled segmental fashion. After several repeats, taking care to come up slowly with the tummy pulled in, her spine felt looser. It would pay out more and grow longer each time, so she could hang there comfortably, dropping lower with each breath.

To increase the control and confidence in the tipping forward and hauling up action, I interspersed the forward bending with rapid curl ups on the couch. These had to be done faster but carefully, without letting the back 'rick'. After doing it successfully (it takes concentration) her trunk control improved dramatically. Not only could she sit up unaided after completing the curl ups but she could put one leg to the floor from the bed and then the other while automatically controlling the spine with her tummy. (She did it while talking, without even thinking.)

A less fit patient takes longer to get to this phase. I always insist people try to get up spontaneously from lying on their backs instead of turning on their sides and pushing up with the hands. This may have been a habit of many years but it will always hamper progress. If practical use is not made immediately of muscles which have been strengthened by formal exercises (the curl ups) they will never get properly strong. It is no use exercising like mad and then never using the newfound power(!)

Georgie was dispatched home to include in her regimen the faster curl ups at the end of the slow, and then to follow these by relaxed forward bending to touch her toes. This program was to be followed at two hourly intervals throughout the day in a special exercise session which also included the loosening preamble of oscillating the knees and pivoting on the lower spine. If her back started to get touchy, she was to lie down for half an hour after exercising.

At other points in the day she was to drop down and squat wherever she was. I specifically asked her to do this whenever she felt the back getting tired and stiff. She was to deliberately break up the gathering castness and not worry about the stretching discomfort this caused. In other words, she should push it aside before it pushed her. (She should bear this in mind for the rest of her life.)

At this stage, Georgie completely took over her own treatment and kept herself totally symptom free. However, I asked her to return four weeks later to beef up her strengthening regime from vertical intrinsics exercises to horizontal ones. Although the vertical intrinsics (the toe touches) are more functional and therefore a more useful form of the exercise, they have a much shorter leverage and are not as strengthening. Exercising them horizontally through a longer leverage also hastens the return of a proper undulating action of spine bending. They are best done off the end of a treatment couch or some other stable surface, like a sturdy kitchen table.

It is often difficult to find somewhere to do this exercise at home. Some people join a gymnasium (Georgie did) where there is an apparatus designed for this purpose (although it is mostly used incorrectly with people flipping up instead of unfurling). At a push you can do the exercise over the back of a sofa, over banisters or a garden rail, provided it is strong enough and the hip bones are protected by a pillow.

Georgie shimmied forward off the front of the treatment couch to the level of her two hip bones while I held her legs. I placed a pillow over her calves and then rested all my weight on her to counter-balance her when she took her hands off the floor. To start, I asked her to fold her arms across her chest and lower her trunk down to 90 degrees, so her hair dragged on the floor.

From this position, I asked her to unfurl to the horizontal position with a wave-like motion along the spine, starting at the base with her head coming up last. She then reversed the action and returned to the floor. Once there, I asked her to hang and relax, particularly the gluteal muscles. On the way up again, I asked her to emphasise the tightening of her buttocks and lower tummy, making the lower torso into a flexible cylinder straightening from the bent over position, like a child's tubular party whistle which uncurls and flings itself out straight when it is blown into.

Because of her general fitness Georgie found this exercise relatively easy, although by the time she had repeated it ten or twelve times she was fairly beat (some people can only do two or three). However, this exercise must not be done too early in recovery. Despite its effectiveness at strengthening the spine it causes marked treatment soreness and the back feels uncomfortable for days. For this reason, I asked Georgie to repeat the exercise no more than two or three times a week, depending on the irritability of her back.

7 Treating your own back

This chapter discusses all the procedures involved in treating your own back. It explains the rationale behind each one and what it will do for you. It also spells out the dos and don'ts of each procedure, and the common pitfalls of each one.

HELPING YOURSELF

With self treatment, it goes without saying that there is no input from anyone else's hands. Although I strongly suggest that in the beginning you see a physiotherapist, manual therapist, chiropractor or osteopath who will isolate your problem and initiate the un-jamming process, the rest of it is up to you. There are many operators who are expert at undoing complex jamming of vertebral segments, but they alone cannot deliver you from trouble. You need to help yourself—and be confident about doing so. Even the best therapeutic magician, who plays the spine with the finesse of a concert pianist, can only address the 'hands on' aspect of your care. The background decompression of your spine and the restoration of your trunk control can only be done by you.

Spinal therapies which do not recruit the sufferer share short-lived success. Yet most people would love to help fix their problem, if only they knew how. A quick tweak here and another tweak there, and a repeat appointment in a couple of weeks, rarely achieves anything if there is no groundwork from you in the meantime. The regenerative period may be a fraction of the degenerative one, yet it still takes time. It is a journey which must methodically unfold as it stops the destruction and turns it around. A condition which has taken years to evolve cannot be cured in a moment, especially when the factors which brought it about (gravity and our upright stance) never go away.

You have to decompress your spine. No-one else can do this for you. You also may have to loosen contracture of the spine's soft tissues. No-one else can do that for you. You have to restore strength to weak muscles. No-one can do this for you either. So except for the subtle art of manually loosening a spinal segment, which is hard for you to execute with any degree of accuracy, you do the vast bulk of rehabilitation yourself. And remember, you have the invaluable advantages of intuition and instinct guiding you from the inside.

The fundamentals of self treatment are to minimise the compression and restore elasticity to an immobile link. This is achieved by stretching your spine, maintaining the vertebral separation, and then going after even more. Minimising vertical compression allows the disc to suck in water which makes it more resilient. Thus it absorbs shock better, so it suffers less trauma. A properly hydrated disc also spares the facet surfaces excessive contact. It acts like a pivot on which the segment tips, while the intrinsic muscles at the back control the forward nodding of the vertebra like horse's reins—all of them working at their most efficient angle of pull. As the disc flattens, there is less of this see-sawing action, and everything works less well. Strain and eventually pain sets in. Restoration of disc height is thus the first objective of treatment. The key to the cure is as simple as knowing the cause.

Preliminary thoughts

Self treatment of a spinal problem involves graduated combinations of a few simple exercises, rather than a great variety. And because the central jamming is the first disorder from which other conditions flow, the fundamentals of all treatments are just the same—even for more complex disorders. The same few exercises keep cropping up: rocking the knees to the chest, spinal rolling, squatting, using the BackBlock, the tennis ball, the Ma Roller, abdominal strengthening exercises (curl ups), toe touches, diagonal toe touches, floor twists and intrinsics exercises.

But before these start, it is important to know that treatment of any problem must be taken at the right rate. In what is essentially a healing process, the regimen must be embarked upon with determination, subtlety and intuition. There should be a fine balancing act between rigour and rest. It has to mean business but cannot be rushed. You have to do what is necessary, unflinchingly, but you cannot harry your back. You must tailor treatment to your spine's ability to recuperate after each 'new' activity.

Be guided by your instincts. You do have to keep pushing the spine at times when you might be fearful about it but remember, most pains are good pains and most people are fearful of the wrong wrongs. They are too defensive and too ready to brace against the pain, wrapping it up, clenching around it and keeping it inside the spine.

It is surprising how dramatically you can reduce your discomfort by willing the muscles around the pain in your back to relax. You can do it during any activity: walking along, waiting for a lift, or stretching to make a bed. As you feel the muscles start to grab, concentrate on making them let go, like a meaningful glance to stop a naughty dog jumping up. Subtle as it is, a breakthrough like this is a huge milestone in the management of your own back problem.

When self treatment fails, it is often because you have been too tense to disengage from the pain. At the same time, there may have been too little or too much physical effort. You may not have been sufficiently calm and persevering or you may have been too vigorous, with too high an expectation of an instant cure. Alternatively, it may have been progressed too recklessly. The clue with self treatment is to keep going, quietly yet purposefully: not too timid, not too aggressive. Just keep going with sensitivity.

Chances are, you will occasionally lose control of the treatment. You will have a hiccup in progress when everything seemed to be going smoothly; a savage twinge as if your back has turned around and bitten you. You will be cast into despair and lose your serene overview, and your confidence will waver. More importantly, you will stop dead. You will not know what has happened and you will be too frightened to keep going. But if you grind to a halt, the back will have taken over again.

Rest assured that at some stage, *all* of you will have to deal with some kind of wobble in the smooth path of recovery. You will think you are getting nowhere; that it shouldn't be this painful. You may feel weak or nauseated or sorer than yesterday. There may be newer pains higher up, or a different type of pain in the same area of your back.

Keep calm and ride out the storm. Employ all the resources you have to avoid panic. Your back is simply complaining about the new rules, and it is very important not to succumb. You need to ease up for a day or so, *but do not stop*. Remember you are on a one-way trip, and the direction is forward. Having stirred up the very centre of things, it is critical to keep going so that in the end there is something to show for it after the reaction has died down.

You will not reach this point if you abort part-way through. You will be left with the sense that whatever you did made you worse. You will have provoked the root cause into an angry reaction lasting several weeks, even months, without the follow-through to see any appreciable gain at the end.

THE PROCEDURES

Bed rest

Sometimes a back problem is too inflamed for exercises to start. When this is the case, the ideal approach is to rest in bed with medication, doing bouts of exercise throughout the day.

Bed rest simply means going to bed, which is usually hard to do. The adjustment in peoples' lives is never easy and invariably you think there must be an easier way. But to do it properly you simply must rest. Furthermore, you have to give yourself over to the notion of doing nothing, with an attitude of abandon rather than frustration, otherwise you will get nowhere.

With cases of severe inflammation, there can be a build-up of treatment soreness which mimics the original pain. If the condition is chronic, the increase in pain is tolerable, but if the segment is acutely inflamed, it will seem as if the treatment has made you worse. Bed rest lets the dust settle. The peaceful periods between the hard work let the inflammation subside and allow your back to recuperate so therapy can go on.

Bed rest also eliminates the compression of gravity, which, as a first measure, starts the unjamming of the spinal link. This first step usually makes the worst of the pain start to fade. Apart from relieving the local engorgement of the problem link, the horizontal resting eases the spasm of the spinal muscles. As they relax, the pain eases as the circulation picks up. There is better natural sluicing of toxic inflammatory products away from the local nerve endings and the pain is no longer ever-present. As the protective spasm eases, the restorative process gathers pace.

The correct way to rest in bed

The important thing about bed rest is that it must be horizontal. It is not as effective on the sofa. You can get up from your bed to shower and get dressed but you must go straight back to bed and stay there, perhaps for several days.

Use a pillow only under your head, two at the most. Avoid using a stack of pillows so that your back hangs in a deep slump. If you are very uncomfortable even lying there, you should have one pillow under your head and several pillows under your lower legs so that the hips and knees are as close to a right angle as possible. This reduces the pressure on your low back.

While you are lying on the bed, try to keep active. Don't lie there rigid because that is the opposite of what you are trying to achieve. Keep relaxed and mobile but always flat, filling your time with the exercises shown below. Rest any way you are comfortable (although all positions become uncomfortable after too long and you will have to move). Gather all your things about you: telephone, books and chairs where people can sit. Your back needs time and peace, so sign off and enjoy the rest.

Take care when getting up. You will have to roll yourself over to the edge of the bed and swing your legs over the side. To lever yourself up sideways, you will have to push into the bed with both arms, with your tummy braced.

Your legs will go down to the floor as your trunk comes up. You should only get up two or three times per day.

Medication

Taking tablets is as unpopular as bed rest. People are wary of entering an arrangement which may have no limits. But in the way that going to bed interrupts the chaos of running a life through pain, taking medication can allow you the space to regroup and soften your mind-set about your back. By surrendering to the very foreigness of taking tablets you may also free yourself from all your previous, rigidly held dictums. Medication, particularly muscle relaxants, helps wipe the slate clean to set a new course in the self management of your problem. By allowing a drug-induced reprieve from feeling your pain and thinking about your problem (which is often more important), medication lays the groundwork for the calm and focused dawning of a new era. Appropriately prescribed medication, in combination with physical influences, can be just what you need to get you over the worst.

The three different categories of medication are painkillers, muscle relaxants and non-steroidal anti-inflammatory drugs (NSAIDS) and they must be prescribed by your medical practitioner.

Painkillers and NSAIDS

The choice of painkiller and anti-inflammatory drugs needs to be discussed with your doctor. He or she will know from your medical history if there are any contra-indications to taking them and will be familiar with features of the different drugs. Getting rid of pain is the main objective so the more powerful the painkiller the better, but it should be for a limited period only and you will need your doctor to supervise. Tablets should be taken three times per day—morning, noon and night—so that the pain is kept at bay at all times. The less pain there is, the less the body reacts to it. (There are many painkillers on the market but be aware that ones with a codeine base cause constipation which can make backpain worse.)

NSAIDS also come in many different forms with brand names like Naprosyn, Voltaren, etc. Their role is to target and actively quell the inflammatory process which is the ultimate source of pain. Under the blanket cover of less pain, they allow the part to keep working normally, but more importantly, they allow more vigorous treatment. NSAIDS should not be taken flippantly. They irritate the bowel and cause nausea, but they must be taken consistently over a set period of time because their effectiveness depends on maintaining a certain level in the blood. They should always be taken with food to reduce their noxious effects.

In a sense, treatment irritates the tissues. It provokes an inflammatory response from all the tugging and stretching to get a segment going again, which brings it to the very brink of what it can take. Treatment is designed to artificially irritate a problem to bring the blood rushing, but in doing this, it walks a tightrope between coaxing the body along at a rate it can accept and overwhelming it with inflammatory reaction. Treatment amounts to 'tailored movement' with all the knockabout excesses of everyday activity smoothed out. But it can also swamp the joint, especially if it is semi-immersed with inflammation to start with. If you are not careful you can develop an acute treatment reaction on top of the underlying chronic one; additional 'man-made' inflammation with more pain on top of the pre-existing lot.

Sometimes the reaction can be so severe, it feels as if the treatment has made you worse. Usually even the worst reactions leave you better off in the long run, although this is often hard to believe at the time. It takes some convincing that all the 'new' pain has anything going for it at all. Provided you do not lock up too much with muscle spasm when the going gets rough (which *can* cause you to be worse off afterwards), the degree of treatment reaction is usually directly proportional to the amount of gain. Furthermore, it actually *helps* at the time to see all the soreness and newfound fragility in your back as a good sign. It helps too when you recognise (which you often can, if you keep clear-headed enough) that the treatment reaction has a different quality to it, so the new pain is actually different from the old one. All these are good signs, although the discomfort nevertheless has to be worked through.

Even so, it is better still to minimise the pain at the start; to knock the peak of it off at the source, to stop the cycle gearing up. Better to take the medication in the expectation that treatment will almost certainly cause a reaction. Better to keep it under wraps, so that when you emerge from the end of treatment with proper function restored, it is like a fog lifting. You stop the medication as the pain fades, and walk free from the rigours of treatment and the anxiety of taking pills.

Muscle relaxants

For various reasons the muscles can take over and make things worse. Sometimes fear alone is sufficient to do this, but at other times the inflammation is so intense, the muscles go into protective mode as part of the spiralling reaction. Muscle spasm is a normal phenomenon when there is pain. However, the degree of spasm for a given level of joint irritability varies widely from one person to the next. It depends on many factors, not least personality type and the presence or absence of other emotional stresses in one's life— some of which may be buried in the subconscious.

It is no overstatement to say that muscle spasm alone can transform a nuisance problem into a tragedy. If it takes hold it can cause things to slide so far that the back can become incurable. Muscle spasm is the wild card with backs. Its bad feature is that it may keep on keeping on, long after the original cause for it has gone away. In other words, it can be the sole stimulus which keeps the inflammatory cycle going. The clenched muscles are painful in themselves (as is any muscle suffering low-grade cramp) but their continuous clench stops blood passing freely though the part. There is pain because the muscle fibres are working overtime and because there is not enough oxygen for their needs.

Muscle spasm is often interwoven with anxiety and depression about the problem which is enough to keep the cycle going—and it is for this reason that muscle relaxants have a role to play. The easing of the muscle hold, even though chemically induced, can break the nexus between pain and reaction-to-pain and create a vital breathing space for recovery.

Muscle relaxants ease muscle spasm, whether that spasm is caused by fear or has an organic origin. Diazepam, otherwise known as Valium, is the best, although it is not without detractors. When your back cannot admit any local movement without a nasty growl of pain, Valium dissolves the grip of the muscles (although it makes you quite stupid in the head). Valium is both addictive and cumulative and needs to be taken under the strict guidance of your doctor so it doesn't become a problem in itself. Its best use is with the first glimmer of an old pain returning. If you have ricked your back and it feels stiff with the first signs of pain down the leg, one Valium and an early night's sleep is often enough to see it off.

At the height of an acute episode the dose should be high enough to cause drowsiness. The ideal amount is 5 mg three times a day (one on rising, one at midday and one after dinner at night). It should make you want to be in bed, docile and floppy like a rag doll so your spine can ease apart at its painful crimped links. It should be enough that when the episode has passed, you cannot recall the sequence of events or the days passing. It can be tailed off once the mobilising is well in train and the initial treatment pain has passed.

EXERCISES FOR TREATING A BAD BACK

Once the stage is set with adequate rest and any necessary drug therapy, the following exercises reverse the structural and functional changes of the motion segment. Basic theoretical treatment regimens, using various combinations of the exercises for specific back disorders, are in Chapters 2 to 6.

Rocking the knees to the chest

The least taxing and therefore least frightening exercise in the early loosening of a jammed segment is rocking the knees to the chest. It is performed in the horizontal supine position to eliminate compression of the spine.

The primary function of the knee rocking exercise is to fan open the posterior compartments of the spine like flaring out a deck of cards. The action stretches the muscles down the back of your spine when their tonic hold has pulled the interspaces shut. Releasing the muscles un-jams the facets and releases the pincer effect on the intervertebral disc. Thus the passive stretching inhibits the additional closing down effect across the inflamed vertebral segment. By providing 'active' decompression it provides the first glimmer of the spine lifting off the compressed segments. It is a very efficient first base exercise.

Like spinal rolling which you will read about below, rocking the knees to the chest is very effective if you have just jarred your spine or hurt it in some way. Rocking has an immediate neuro-physiological 'switching off' effect which defuses the alarm and pre-empts the local muscles locking up the spine. The to-and-fro rocking action familiarises your back with movement again so it doesn't have time to get stiff. It keeps your back moving in a non-threatening way and encourages the fundamental physiologies—unhindered blood flow and proper drainage—to resume.

In the acute phase the pull-and-release evacuates the inflammatory products from the site of injury. With more chronic conditions, the main benefit is the physical stretching of the tight structures. The non-weight-bearing loosening of all the soft tissues of the posterior compartment, including the back wall of the disc, immediately gives the tight segment more freedom to move.

Although rocking the knees to the chest is most effective for segmental stiffness of L5 and L4, it is also effective higher up in the lumbar spine where there may be some rotation of the segment as well.

Simple as it sounds, rocking the knees is often difficult to get started, let alone do well. If your back is in acute distress it is not easy to get the knees to the chest. Your legs feel heavy and your spine is loathe to bend, and you may get stabs of pain as you grapple with lifting your thighs. As the spine starts to round more easily, your hip joints often complain about being bunched onto the chest. It may be more comfortable for the hips if you allow your knees to part widely around the abdomen. (You may also may find that one leg is more comfortable doing this movement than the other.)

With the more chronic disorders, where your lower back may have been stiff for decades, the cement-like rigidity is often unwilling to yield. The lower segments move as a rigid block, with all the hinging taking place at the hips and the upper lumbar levels. As the segments ease apart, your back starts to round more easily, making it a natural progression to spinal rolling, which is discussed below.

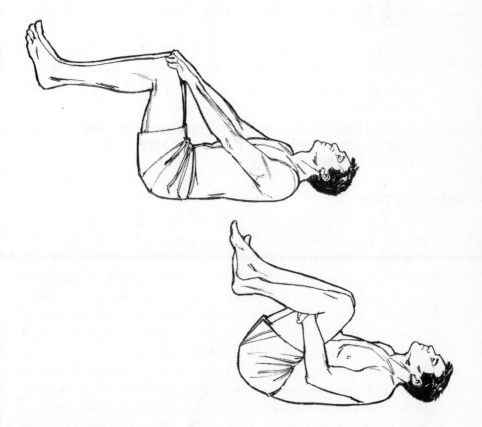

Figure 7.1 Rocking the knees to the chest

The emphasis with rocking the knees is to keep the movement as subtle as possible. Don't be tempted to tug at your knees with the muscles in your neck standing up. Don't jab your head up to meet the knees. Leave your head and shoulders calm and relaxed on the floor and gently oscillate your legs with the fingers interlaced around both knees. As your back relaxes a sense of movement will dawn, like a piece of frozen meat thawing. The tightness will fade as you feel the vertebrae gapping open at the back. Don't hurry and try to imagine the vertebrae segments pulling apart.

THE CORRECT WAY OF ROCKING THE KNEES TO THE CHEST

- Lie on your back on the bed or on a soft surface on the floor.

- Brace your low back by sucking your navel in hard. If your tummy is weak, push in with one hand on the front of the tummy for reinforcement.

- With the other hand behind your thigh, pull one leg up to the chest. As soon as one foot is off the bed you can use both hands to pull the leg on to the chest.

- Bracing your tummy in the same way, pull the other leg onto your chest and cross both ankles.

- Cup a hand over each knee and then move your legs so the thighs rest at 90°. Oscillate gently in this position.

- For high lumbar problems, take your knees lower down to the chest, let the ankles cross and link your wrists across the upper shins, below the knees. Oscillate in this position.

Spinal rolling

Spinal rolling is important in self treatment. It breaks up the superficial brittleness of the column and is the simplest form of spinal mobilisation. Each vertebra has its turn at gliding past its neighbours as your bodyweight rolls over it. Again using the analogy of the keyboard, rolling along the spine is like rolling your forearm and wrist down over an expanse of piano keys as they depress one after the other. Instead of sounding a different musical note, each vertebra has its own note of stiffness, although the jammed one is especially shrill as your bodyweight passes over it.

In this regard, rolling along the spine is a primitive diagnostic tool. By rolling over the segments you can isolate your problem level. You can 'examine' the L4–L5 and the lumbo-sacral interspaces by clasping your hands behind your knees and nearly straightening your legs with toes high in the air. The weight of the legs and the long leverage make it easy for you to tip back and forth over the lower end of the spine to see whether you elicit pain. To isolate the mid-lumbar level, hug your knees a little closer to the chest so that they make a shorter lever. Depending on the bulk of the upper chest, the angle at the knees will be closer to a right angle. To isolate the thoraco-lumbar level, you have to shorten the lever even more by having your legs pointing almost straight up to the ceiling. To tip your weight towards the higher end of the lumbar spine, you simply bend and straighten your knees in the air, which rocks the body back and forth.

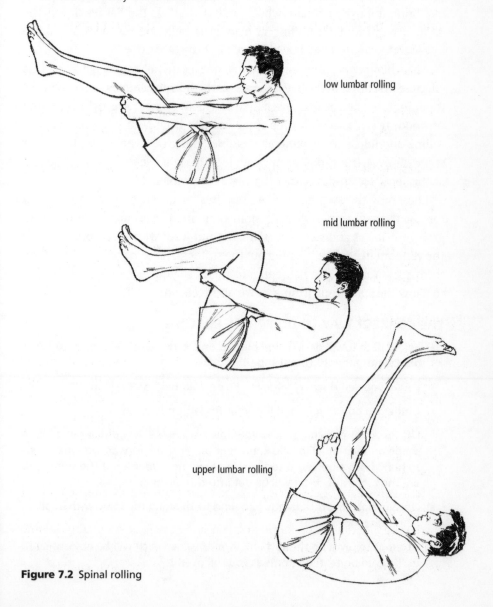

low lumbar rolling

mid lumbar rolling

upper lumbar rolling

Figure 7.2 Spinal rolling

All these movements require a fair degree of control and will not be possible in phases of acute pain. Simple as they sound, it is often too painful to get your spine rounded sufficiently and you struggle about stranded, like a beetle on its back.

Or it may not be painful at all, simply stiff. The patch of immobility may be loathe to press out the other way because the vertebrae cannot glide backwards. (I can see this as a small hollow scoop in the low back when you bend forward from the standing position.) It makes rolling along the spine like bumping over a square wheel, with a clonk as the flat patch hits the floor. It requires extra pulling in below the belly button to shrink in the lower abdomen, to force the stiff patch out the other way.

As a therapeutic exercise, spinal rolling is the all-round panacea. It is effective first thing in the day if there is early morning stiffness. It also breaks the spine free of guarding muscle spasm which can hold it as rigid as a plank of wood. It is also useful if the spine has just been jarred; in this case, the rolling should be as relaxing as possible, along the whole length of your spine. As everything loosens up, your legs tip right back over your head and as the spine softens it is easier to isolate the problem level.

Loosening the specific vertebra requires small range pivoting back and forth with small amplitude excursions right on the painful spot. You have to grab your knees and steer yourself back and forth with precision. Working the vertebra free is like pressing out the stiffness, pivoting back and forth on the carpet. You can also pause in mid-flight, staying motionless on the spot to allow the spine time to sink down and relax around it.

THE CORRECT WAY TO DO SPINAL ROLLING

- Fold a bath towel double and place it on a carpeted area of floor to roll on. Do not attempt to roll in bed.

- Lower yourself down carefully to lie on your back on the floor.

- Gather up both thighs and link your fingers under them.

- Lift up your head and neck so your low back makes a wide rounded 'U' shape on the floor. (To help keep your upper trunk forward you may need to bend both elbows out to the side as you hold your legs.) The stiffer you are the more difficult it will be get into this position.

- Once in position, rock gently back and forth along the spine with small amplitude movements.

- Attempt to pivot on the stiff link in your spine which will be obvious by its 'bruised bone' tenderness as you roll over it.

- Use your legs for leverage. As you straighten them out they alter your weight distribution and make it easier to tip towards the lower end of the spine. If you keep your legs bunched up on your chest it will focus the rolling towards the upper end of the spine and require more jerking effort of your head to bring it down to the lower end.

- Continue for 15–30 seconds, trying to relax as much as possible as you do it. Let the gentle rocking motion mesmerise you.

- To rest, put one foot on the floor, and then the other, leaving both knees crooked. Do not put your legs down flat.

- Resume at one minute intervals and repeat up to five times.

- This is not an easy exercise to overdo. Cramp of the tummy muscles may be the only thing that stops you.

Curl ups

Tummy muscles play an important role in off-loading the base of the spine. They do this by co-contracting with the back muscles which tenses the abdominal cylinder and raises the abdominal pressure. This lifts the spine skywards and increases the tension between the vertebral links. Strong tummy muscles also control the way the vertebrae move during upright activity. They help the vertebrae to tip forward rather than shear when the spine bends. Thus tummy strength plays a critical role in optimal spinal performance.

For this reason, curl ups are probably the single most important exercise in the prevention and management of spinal problems. In short, they not only prevent the spine harming itself but, once a spine *is* in trouble, they help get the segments back to full function.

However, if curl ups are done badly, as a flipping-up action with a straight back, you will impact the segments and make them shear. This explains the painful tweak you can get jerking up aggressively. You must *never* come up with a straight back, angling at the hips with your belly distending like a beach ball to be struggled around. If your back clicks or hurts as you do curl ups, pull your tummy in harder and round your lower back more.

Good curl ups must incorporate the oblique muscles (which pull in the sides of the waist) as well as the transversus abdominus muscle (which pulls in below the navel). You should be able to see the small diagonal slips of the external oblique muscles standing out through the skin at the sides of the chest wall. If you are weak, the best way to incorporate transversus abdominus is on the return journey to the floor. Keeping your back round, you should press the whole lumbar area into the floor and lower one vertebra at a time.

Never hinge back and forth in mid-air using the strong muscles of the hips (iliopsoas) and keeping your spine straight. Always go right up and right down, putting your head down last, like a roll of carpet being rolled up and rolled out across the floor. Also, never do tummy exercises in the way of the popular 'crunches'. These do exactly what they say: telescope the spine into its base, crunching the lower vertebrae together. Crunches also over-use the upper abdominals and under-use the lower ones. Done to excess they cause a shoulders-hunched posture and a paunchy pot-belly below the navel. Even as you do crunches, you can feel the overwork in the wrong place— strain over the front of the rib cage while the low belly stays poking out.

When a low back is painful, curl ups play an important neuro-physiological role in reducing the hold of the back muscles. When worked strongly they automatically make the long back muscles switch off. This simple-is-genius truism of physiology is a very effective way of making a stiff back relax. Curl ups also reduce stiffness simply because the long back muscles have to stretch around the rounded prominence of the low back. The elongation of your spine (especially if you continue forward through your knees with your head down) stretches and softens their muscular clench and allows the spinal segments to ease apart.

THE CORRECT WAY TO DO CURL UPS

- Lying on your back with your knees bent and the front of your feet wedged under a sofa or a bed, bring your chin to your chest with both arms outstretched over your knees.

- Hump your lower back, pressing it into the floor.

- Roll along the dish-shaped low back and, without jerking, curl up to a sitting position. If the initial effort is too great then pull lightly with the hands behind the thighs to roll yourself up.

- Go past the sitting position and then, by parting your knees, go through the legs until the whole spine is curled fully forward into a stretch, head down. Keep your tummy sucked in.

- The return to the floor is more important and requires full control, without hanging on to the thighs. Keep your belly sucked in like a greyhound, nipped in below the navel.

- Tip the pelvis back, press the lumbar spine into the floor to make a crease across your belly and roll down along the spine like unrolling a carpet.

- Repeat at least 15 times for every one minute on the BackBlock. For getting rid of muscle spasm or for pure strengthening, this number must increase dramatically.

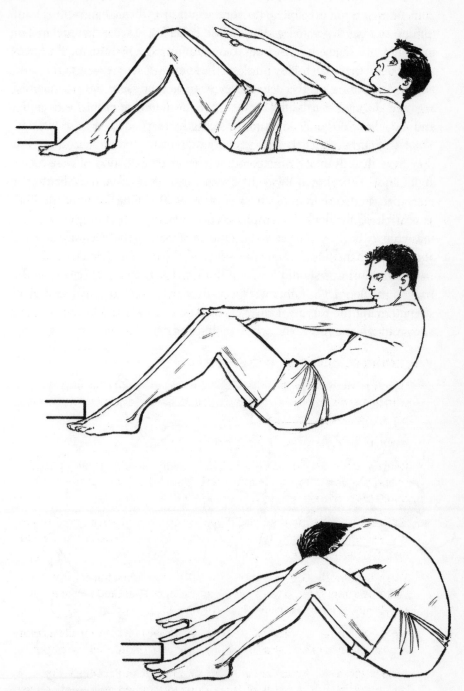

Figure 7.3 Curl ups

Reverse curl ups

Sometimes it is not possible to do normal curl ups when strengthening your tummy. In cases of severe leg pain (caused either by an acute disc prolapse or instability of a segment) it is better to do tummy work by bringing the knees to the chin rather than rolling up along the spine. Because reverse curl ups do not involve sitting on the pelvis, they exert less pressure on the inflamed segment and are less irritating for the nerve. High lumbar problems (from L3 and above) also do better with tummy strengthening done as reverse curl ups.

Reverse curl ups are relatively strenuous compared to normal curl ups but they have the advantage of demanding greater participation of transversus abdominus. They should always be done lying on the back and oscillating the knees back and forth from a starting position of 90°, lifting the bottom as high as possible off the floor. The emphasis should be on knees to the chin rather than chin to the knees. Never start the movement lifting the feet from the floor, and returning them back there; the weight of the legs can strain the back.

Reverse curl ups should be done if normal curl ups hurt (either in the back, buttock or leg). In many respects they are a less problematical way of strengthening the tummy. However, they do not have the benefit of your body rolling along your spine, which mobilises a rigid mass of spinal segments.

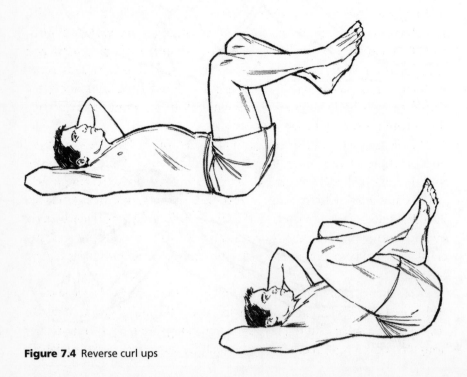

Figure 7.4 Reverse curl ups

THE CORRECT WAY TO DO REVERSE CURL UPS

- Lie on your back on the floor and take first one knee onto your chest, then the other.

- Crossing the feet at the ankles and letting the knees fall apart comfortably, take the thighs to 90°, and interlace your fingers behind your neck.

- By lifting your bottom clear of the floor use your tummy to bring your knees up under your chin.

- At the same time, bring your chin to meet your knees and hold them there momentarily.

- As you relax and your legs come down, make sure they do not pass beyond 90° which would cause your back to arch.

- When you get into your stride, you can swing your knees up with some gusto, as long as you do not jar your back.

- Repeat fifteen times.

Using the BackBlock

Used under both the upper back and the sacrum, the BackBlock straightens and decompresses the spine. Apart from pulling the segments apart it re-establishes the spine's proper 'S' bends. If the back is too stooped it straightens it. In the thoracic area it opens out a round-shouldered look, and at the keystone of the spine—the base—it pushes the bottom in and straightens the entire skeleton. On the other hand, if the low back is too hollow, it can reverse that too. Lying passively over the BackBlock, the vertebrae inch backwards and the high arch of the lumbar area slowly drops flatter towards the floor.

The BackBlock is also the natural antidote to sitting, which we Westerners do all the time. Placed under the sacrum and the thorax in turn, it prises out the hours of slumped 'C'-shaped compression and stretches out the tightness of your hips and knees which have also spent so much time bent. Thus the BackBlock uses gravity to press your spine straighter, aligning it more trimly over its narrow base. In this way it deals with its two main pain-making causes at once: basal compression and the spine's dynamic imbalance over the sacrum.

Although our nearest cousins the apes have a rounded 'C'-shaped stature, with their heads carried well forward, in front of the line of gravity, they can reverse any problems this might cause by swinging through the trees on their arms (brachiating). Human beings have no such means of traction to straighten their spines, and must counter the ill-effects all their lives. Most of us have to work at keeping a good posture and decompressing our bases otherwise we get low backpain. A BackBlock, nothing more than a simple chunk of wood, is a most effective tool.

When the BackBlock pulls apart the lumbar segments it creates a negative suction effect which drags fluids from the vertebral bodies into the disc. The stretching also makes the stiffened disc walls more pliable, so it is easier for the colloidal jelly of the disc's nucleus to exercise its phenomenal pull on water to expand and fill the space. With more room to move between the separated vertebrae, both suction and attraction forces work together to make a much quicker job of hydrating the discs. In no time, they become fluid-filled and bursting to make better shock absorbers.

You must always start off using the BackBlock on its flattest side. As your legs drop down and you feel the pelvis pulling off the base of your spine you often feel a tug in your back, right where it hurts. It feels as if it really means business; as if a screwdriver is boring right into your pain. At first it may take some concentration to relax and let the discomfort fade. Some people take several weeks to progress to the middle height of the BackBlock, while others go straight to it. Nobody should attempt to use it on end first off. Initially you must remain on the Block no longer than a minute. It is better to do repeated short sessions than one long one. If you stay there too long it can be difficult to get off. There is always a murmur of discomfort as you lift your bottom off the Block, and if you have been there too long, what should be a little pain becomes a big pain. Although this will not harm you in the long run, it can be unnerving. Better to do shorter sessions, followed by the usual rocking the knees to the chest and curl ups after the BackBlock has been removed.

It is imperative to *always* follow the BackBlock with curl up exercises. After rocking the knees has first removed the castness of your back, and got it used to humping round the other way, you should go straight to curl ups. If you progress to staying longer on the Block (say up to two or three minutes, which you must only do when you have become a dab hand at it), you must always increase the number of curl ups proportionately. If you fail to do enough curl ups when using the Block (or worse still none at all) your back will feel very stiff and sore over the next few days. Curl ups and the BackBlock should be balanced, otherwise the benefit is reduced. If people are sore after using the Block, they have invariably forgotten their curl ups.

The BackBlock is a dream to use under your upper back. Apart from taking the hunch out of your spine it makes you feel taller and your body looser in its skin, especially when you take your arms over your head, linking fingers and turning the palms away. You can feel your whole spine pulling out of your pelvis like a cobra out of its basket with a beautiful emancipating stretch which goes right from your chest through to your waist and low back. The BackBlock should be placed on its flattest side, lengthways under the long curve of the thoracic spine, so the top edge is level with the top of your shoulders and the lower edge at high waist level (sometimes, if you are short, it digs in here until you loosen up over the next couple of days). As you lie back, you may need to lower your head back to the floor with your hands and when there, elongate the back of your neck by pulling your chin in. Some people feel nauseated on first putting their head back, but this passes as they get used to it.

To help reverse the pinched-forward look of the shoulders which so often goes with a stooped upper back, you can stretch the pectoral muscles at the front of the chest by moving your arms as you lie back over the BackBlock. Chest expansion and ease of breathing is also enhanced if you do these actions in time with your respiration. Inhale as you move your arms out from your sides in a large semicircle, to above your head, keeping the back of the hands in contact with the carpet all the way up. For the return journey, exhale as you bring your arms back down to your sides again.

Both ways, the arms will lift off the floor when they approach the 'eagle wings' position in the top quadrant of the semicircle. Through both excursions up and down, there will usually be a stretch across the front of the chest and into the upper arms. To get off the BackBlock when it has been under the thoracic spine you simply roll off to the side like a log. Do not attempt to sit forward because this would strain your neck.

Even though it gets progressively less painful as you repeat each one minute session on the Block, the structural changes take some time to reverse and definite signs of improvement are slower to be realised. Over the first week or so the pain feels less heavy and dull and your back works better. It feels lighter, as if you are no longer dragging an armour-plated shell around with you. Your back feels less blocked and dense with movement; it feels as if the segments are freer to move individually. Especially in a prematurely 'old' and chronically stiff back, these changes and the easing of pain can feel nothing short of miraculous. With more acute problems however, it is less straightforward. Where there is guarding from the muscle spasm, the BackBlock gives better results if it is taken more slowly, and if you have had a bad flare-up you should stop using the Block for two or three days.

Incidentally, you can get the same effect by using a telephone book, or something flatter if you need to. (In cases of acute disc prolapse and acute instability, simply lying flat on your back on the floor brings about the same effects but in a milder way.) A proper BackBlock is better than a miscellany of books because it can be more easily progressed through its various stages: from its lowest side, when the spine is particularly impacted, to the highest side when the spine is in its final stages of rehabilitation. Apart from its stringent dimensions, it also serves as a neat and timely reminder as you spy it sitting in the corner by the TV. Just having it there makes you more likely to use it. And the BackBlock really comes into its own with travelling. All the carrying of heavy luggage, plus the long hours spent sitting and sleeping on unfamiliar beds means that you often need it most when you are away from home. They are hollow, so they are light to transport.

THE CORRECT WAY TO USE THE BACKBLOCK

- Lie on your back on the floor with knees bent.

- Lift your bottom and slide the BackBlock sideways on its flattest side under the sacrum, the broad flat bone at the base of the spine between the two dimples of either buttock.

- Slowly straighten one leg then the other by sliding the heel out away from you along the floor.

- With both legs straight, relax completely and let the weight of your legs pull the spine out. Attempt to keep your heels close together although the toes can roll out. There is frequently a local discomfort at the base of the spine and higher up if another level is jammed there. You should be able to sense the spine pulling apart longitudinally. It is usually an 'agreeable' discomfort, but it should feel as if it means business. Do not be alarmed by the pain. Go with it.

- If you feel absolutely nothing with the BackBlock on its flattest side, then immediately progress to its middle side with the thin edge transversely across the sacrum. You can experiment with sliding the BackBlock up and down under the sacrum to feel where it is fractionally more comfortable. Where it feels best is where it should be. It must *never* be under the spine itself, where it will be very uncomfortable. (I am often surprised how patients forget and put it here.)

- With the BackBlock at the right height, remain in position for one minute, completely relaxed as the legs imperceptibly drop down.

- After a minute, slowly bend one knee and slide the foot up towards the buttock, then the other.

- Lift your bottom off the BackBlock. This can be painful but is no cause for alarm. Move slowly and keep the tummy braced as you slide the Block out to one side.

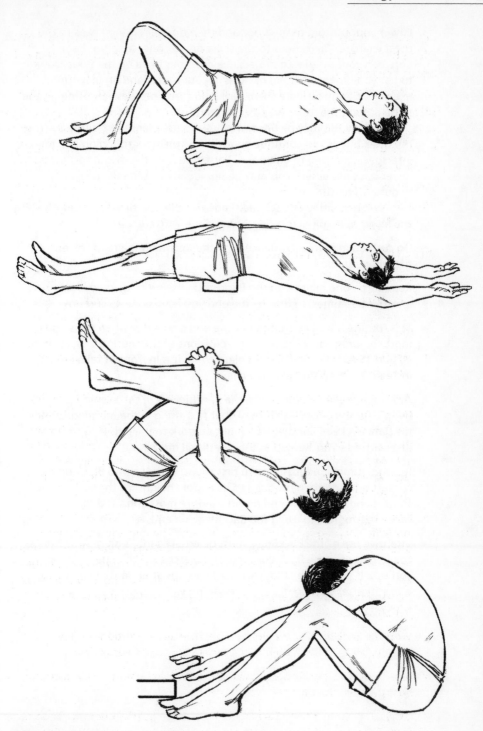

Figure 7.5 BackBlock routine

- Lower your bottom to the floor and then do the rocking knees to the chest exercise. Take knees to the chest one by one, cupping them between your interlaced fingers, leaving your head on the floor. Do not tug at your knees with the muscles in your neck standing up with exertion. Gently oscillate them back and forth, persuasively bringing the spine around the other way into a hump.

  Initially this may be uncomfortable, with a sense of tightness across the base, but as you continue you will feel the back rounding and lower interspaces starting to gap open. Persevere until the discomfort across the lower back has eased. This may be immediate or can take up to two minutes of gentle rocking.

  When your lower back feels more supple, it is time for strengthening the lower abdominal muscles. This is done with curl ups.

- Do curl ups in strict accordance with the instructions already given, fifteen in number.

- Repeat the one minute on the BackBlock, the rocking and curl ups another two times, so that by the end you have done 45 curl ups.

- This routine is best carried out at the end of the day when the spine is most compressed. Three to four repetitions of the routine takes between 10 and 15 minutes and a good place to do it is in front of television, instead of sitting slumped in a chair.

- Although the ideal time to use the BackBlock is in the evening, some people have a better day if they do it first thing in the morning. Some of my patients keep another BackBlock at work to use in the lunch hour after sitting scrunched up at their desks all morning.

- It is sometimes kinder to do the first round with the BackBlock on its flattest side and then progress to its middle height for the second and third round. It takes several months before most impacted spines are ready to progress to using the BackBlock on end.

- Intensive use of the BackBlock must be entered into slowly. At all times, the period over the BackBlock must be matched with equal time doing curl ups. If you use the Block without curl ups afterwards it will be cast and stiff after getting up, and everything will be much more sore and achey.

Using the Ma Roller

The Ma Roller is an effective way of mobilising the chain of facets running down either side of the spine. It looks like a convoluted rolling pin with two large rounded humps either side of a central depression. You position the Roller under the spine, with the row of knobs you can see through the skin over the central gully, and you mobilise the joints either side by rolling up and down as the Roller moves on the floor.

The Ma Roller is more effective under the thoracic spine where the facet joints are nearer the surface (although it hurts more resting your full weight down) but it is still a useful way of isolating and mobilising stiff lumbar facets. As you oscillate back and forth on the painful spot(s), like a bull rubbing against a low branch of a tree, you feel the bitter sweet pain of the stiff joints being worked.

To specifically target the lumbo-sacral facets you position the Roller just above the two dimples in your low back (you are in the right spot when it hurts more) and hump and hollow your low back in a pelvic rocking action over the Roller. As your back hollows it bends around the prominence of the Roller, letting your bottom reach the floor. As your back muscles relax you can feel the delicious pain of the joints being pushed to their limit of range. You can get better access to a single joint by removing the Roller and re-positioning one end only under the side of your spine. With the other side of your back lying on the floor you get deeper pressure onto the problem joint, although you must take care not to cause bruising as you seek it out.

In mobilising an acutely tender facet, it is better to use a tennis ball instead of a Roller. The softer, more yielding ball is kinder to the joint and minimises the risk of making it sore. A tennis ball is also much easier to carry with you when travelling.

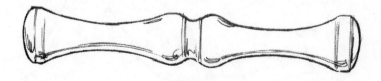

Figure 7.6 The Ma Roller

THE CORRECT WAY TO USE A MA ROLLER

- Lie on your back on carpet with your knees bent and feet flat on the floor.

- Lift your bottom and place the Roller under the midline of your back with the knobs of your spine situated over the central gully of the Roller.

- Raising your upper body with your elbows, gently roll your lower spine up and down over the Roller as it makes small oscillations on the floor.

- The problem joints cause a shriller pain as you pass over them. Stay on these points, 'worrying' them as you travel back and forth.

- To avoid bruising, never spend more than 60 seconds working one joint.

- To remove the Roller, lift your bottom up carefully, taking the Roller out to one side.

- Relax the back by lying down gently on the floor and rocking the knees to your chest for 30 seconds.

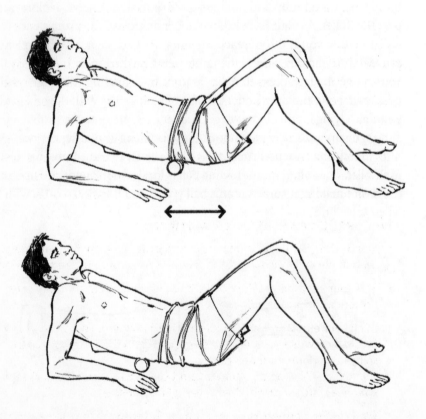

Figure 7.7 Using the Ma Roller

Squatting

Squatting is the natural predecessor to sitting. In an earlier evolutionary state, although we might have run all day holding a spear, at least we squatted around the campfire in the evenings and eased out the compression caused by the day's activity.

Squatting pulls the spinal segments apart and vertically opens the intervertebral spaces from both above and below, rather like extending a tubular fishing net by holding a string at the base with your foot and pulling up the top rim. As the spine elongates, the discs are forced to suck in fluid.

Squatting is also the antidote to sitting. It pulls the segments apart after they have been compressed by the thoracic spine bearing down during lengthy periods perched on the sitting bones. Squatting is the natural partner to the BackBlock. It levers open the back of the disc more while the BackBlock levers open the front, with the result that the entire circumference of the latticed walls is pulled up.

Deep in the squat your knees often complain, but after a week or so they get to love it and you can stay down longer. Keeping your knees wide while squatting and trying to get as much bend as possible at the hips also helps to release tight gluteal muscles which go with low-grade back problems. The more you can force yourself into the extremes of the stretch, the more you break up the overall picture of tightness and the more easily your spine will bend afterwards.

All of us should squat at regular intervals throughout the day, especially after impact activities like running, walking or playing sport. Sometimes you do it instinctively after standing for a long time, when the spine feels a need to break free of the painful castness of spinal compression.

THE CORRECT WAY TO DO SQUATTING

- Stand with your heels and toes close together and, holding the side of the bath or a secure rail, bend the knees and drop your bottom to the floor.

- Part your knees to the limit and without falling backwards take your bottom as close to the floor as possible.

- Bend your elbows to pull yourself forward and drop your head as low as possible between your legs, attempting to turn the full length of the spine into a long, rounded hump.
  In this position gently bounce your bottom to the floor while keeping your head tucked down. Continue for 30 seconds.

- While in this position, suck your tummy in and sense the increase in the separation of the lower segments as the pelvis drops down off the base of the spine.

- To stand up, pull your tummy in and push strongly through the thighs.

- Repeat twice.

- If you do not have a suitable object to hang back from as you squat, you can do it free standing on your haunches. In this position you can sense your spine 'growing' as you pull your tummy in and the back lets go. As your back rounds, you can feel your bottom dropping down closer to the ground.

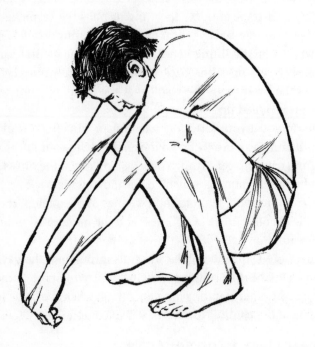

Figure 7.8 Squatting

Toe touches in the standing position

This exercise mimics the longitudinal stretch of squatting and also improves the muscular control of the spine. It stretches shrunken facet capsules and back walls of discs (and the other transvertebral structures). Toe touches improve the coordination and strength of all the muscles which control bending.

Although for years people have been told never to bend if they have a bad back, the benefits of doing so are vast. The deep bend pulls the spine out of its vertical clench and releases the discs to imbibe fluid. It also re-educates the power of the intrinsic muscles which specifically control the tipping of the segments.

Toe touches reduce the overactivity of para-spinal muscles, a common feature of chronically painful backs. They pass the control back to the deeper muscles (the spinal intrinsics and transversus abdominus) so the vertebrae are less likely to shear as the spine bends over.

Toe touches have another important role in the later stages of treatment. Done repetitively and with gusto they plump up the lumbar discs. As the spine rhythmically bends and straightens it creates a fluid exchange through the discs which primes them for optimal performance as core jamming is lifted.

THE CORRECT WAY TO DO TOE TOUCHES

- Stand with the feet 15 cm (6 inches) apart and parallel.

- Contract the buttocks and at the same time pull your tummy in to shrink the circumference of the lower abdomen.

- By tipping your pelvis back slightly so your lower back humps, take your chin onto your chest and curl forward, from the top down, towards the floor.

- Make sure the lower abdomen feels firm and secure, like a tense tube bending with control in the middle.

- Slide both hands down the front of your thighs and on towards the floor.

- If your hamstrings are tight you can bend your knees so you hang there like a gorilla.

- In this position keep the lower abdomen pulled in like a greyhound. Although your tummy will feel pulled in and hard, your lower back should feel a gentle stretching discomfort with a sense of letting go.

- Let your head dangle and your arms flop.

- Try and visualise the bottom vertebrae gapping apart as the bottom of your spine rounds into a hump.

- Without losing the bracing control of the tummy, bounce imperceptibly at the bottom of the bend. The bouncing should be gentle and coaxing, not vigorous. Do several small bounces and then tighten your buttocks in preparation for coming up.

- The return to upright stance has to be done in a controlled way, with the abdomen fully sucked in and the buttocks clenched.

- Come up with an unfurling action, initiated by the pelvis tipping backwards and the rest of the spine following on, the head coming up last.

- In the way that correct curl ups emphasise segmental control, the same is true of toe touches. Especially on the return journey, each vertebra, one after the other, should tip backwards until the upright posture is arrived at.

- Repeat the toe touches three times, trying to get further down with each imperceptible bounce.

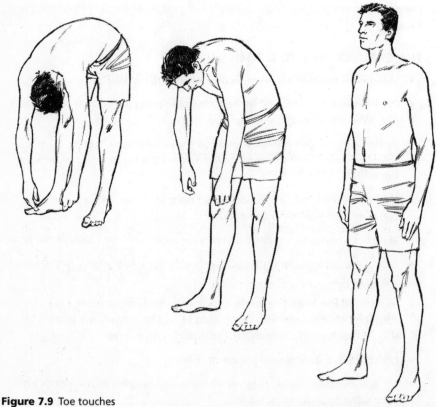

Figure 7.9 Toe touches

Diagonal toe touches

This variation of toe touches comes into its own when treating facet joint problems and chronic disc problems. In the forward bending phase, where you stand with your legs wide apart, taking the left hand down past the right ankle (and vice versa), the capsules of right facet joints are stretched and mobilised. You will always find it is harder bringing your hand to the ankle of the same side as your pain. Thus if you have a right-sided facet problem, it will always be more restricted taking your left hand to the right ankle. The inelastic facet capsule on the right finds it difficult to give out and stretch as the tail of the vertebra swings across to the left.

The return journey to upright position, through the diagonal unfurling movement from the floor, is particularly valuable in strengthening the multi-fidus muscle, usually indicated after a facet locking episode and cases of facet instability. As you come up from taking the left hand past the right ankle, right-sided multifidus pulls on the tail of the vertebra and swings it back towards the midline, thus untwisting the spine. Strengthening this small muscle, which blends so intimately with the facet capsule, helps shore up the joint and makes it less likely to slip out of place. When you have a one-side problem, it is important to repeat the exercise more times to the problem side.

THE CORRECT WAY TO DO DIAGONAL TOE TOUCHES

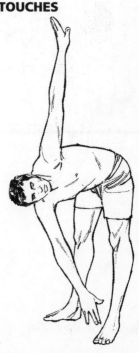

- Stand with your feet 1 metre (3 feet) apart and your hands by your sides.

- Pulling in the tummy hard and clenching the buttocks, bend forward taking the left hand down towards the right ankle.

- If possible, take your hand past the ankle and make small bounces, all the time keeping the tummy pulled in.

- Keeping the hands low, return to the vertical in a diagonal unfurling action, initiated by your buttocks contracting and rolling the pelvis back. Do not take your hands above your head.

- Repeat four times to the problem side to every one to the good side.

Figure 7.10 Diagonal toe touches

Floor twists

This twisting action is done on the floor with the spine unweighted, which puts minimal pressure on the discs as it opens the facet of the underside. Repeating the stretch in the other direction stretches the disc wall the other way and forcibly closes the facets which had previously been gapped.

The twisting stretch of the spine always makes subsequent longitudinal separation much easier and you will notice this yourself when exercising. The spine feels looser to bend after it has twisted both ways first, and you will always get better separation on the BackBlock doing your twists first.

Floor twists also stretch the nerve root where it has become tethered to the inside of the spinal canal or the intervertebral exit canal. Although root sleeve fibrosis is more common after the inflammation of disc prolapse or facet joint arthropathy, it can also exist with loss of disc height through puckering of the intervertebral tissues and the crowding on the nerve.

To get full stretch on the nerve and its rootlets, you have to get proper straightening of the uppermost knee. The same stretch also increases the tension through the hamstrings muscle of the same side. This is valuable because the hamstrings often retain a low level of contraction when there is chronic inflammation of the low lumbar nerve roots. Apart from being a

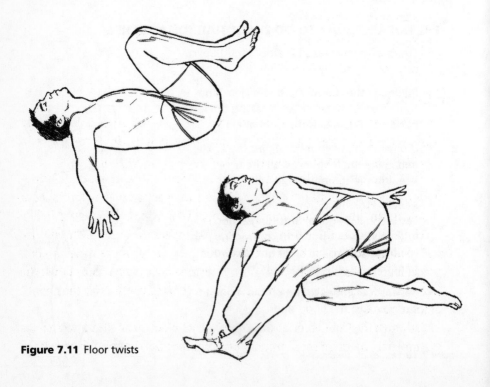

Figure 7.11 Floor twists

mild source of pain in itself, the lack of extensibility of the muscle disturbs the sit of the pelvis and shortens the length of stride of that leg during walking. Both factors exert a subtle background influence on the rate of recovery of the spinal problem.

THE CORRECT WAY TO DO FLOOR TWISTS

- Clear a large uncluttered space on the floor.

- Lie down on your back and bring both knees to the chest, one at a time.

- Place both arms outstretched on the floor at shoulder height with the palms facing the floor.

- Keeping both knees high, let both fall over to the right so the right upper thigh is lying along the floor. As the legs go over, try to prevent the left hand lifting off the floor.

- Make sure that both knees remain as high as possible on the floor with both thighs level, side by side.

- In this position, straighten the top (left) leg at the knee and take hold of the left foot with the right hand. If possible bring the left foot closer to the nose with the right hand.

- Hold for 30 seconds, bouncing the leg minutely by pulling on the toes.

- Repeat to the other side.

- Repeat each way twice.

The Cobra

The Cobra is for stretching—not strengthening. Like curl ups done badly, this exercise can be potentially troublesome if it is done too early in rehabilitation. It comes into its own later on to finish the job.

The Cobra involves lying prone with the palms face down on the floor underneath your shoulders. With a straightening action of the elbows, your shoulders are lifted up and the spine drops passively into a hanging arch.

The action does three things: it forcibly stretches the anterior (front) disc wall and the soft tissue structures spanning the front of the intervertebral space; it compresses the back of the disc; it also maximally closes down the facets at the back of the spine which has a regenerative effect on the growth of joint cartilage.

Although the Cobra seems similar to the BackBlock in its effects, it employs a completely different set of principles. It compresses the spine, whereas the

BackBlock pulls it apart—a fundamental difference between doing the action prone and supine. The exercise increases the arching of the spine, whereas the BackBlock reduces it (although there is a temporary increase initially until the hip flexors lengthen). The Cobra increases the overriding of the facets at the back of the spine whereas through the backward gliding of the vertebrae, the BackBlock disengages the facet surfaces.

The difference in dynamics is profound and this is exactly why the Cobra is so useful—especially in the later stages of treatment when it is used in unison with the BackBlock.

The extreme arching under pressure milks the posterior (back) compartments and helps reduce the swelling of chronically inflamed facets. It also encourages better fluid movement through the discs. Similar to squeezing the rubber knob on the top of a basting tube, you get better suction up the tube if you expel all the air first. The same is true of a stiff and unresponsive motion segment: if it is pressure-evacuated first, you get better separation of both front and back compartments. At the same time, the pressure dints the cartilage covering the facet joint surfaces. As they un-dint, they suck a fluid exchange through the cartilage bed.

The Cobra also keeps the abdominal muscles long. It keeps them from shortening as a result of the vigorous strengthening regimen of sixty or so curl ups per session. Thus the Cobra is a very effective treatment, as long as the segment is not too irritable.

You can beef up the exercise and improve the coordination of the muscles controlling the spine by switching back and forth between the Cobra and the Pose of the Child. This is where you rest your bottom back on your feet and put your forehead on the floor. As you do this, allow your arms to remain stretched out in front of you, draped across the floor. This increases the longitudinal separation through the length of the spine.

THE CORRECT WAY TO DO THE COBRA

- Lie face down on the floor with your legs straight and your hands on the floor beneath your shoulders.

- By straightening the elbows and pushing on the hands, push your upper trunk back off the floor.

- Attempt to straighten the elbows fully but at the same time, try to keep the pubic bone on the floor.

- If you are stiff, let the pelvis lift off the floor so that the body remains suspended. Do not let your hands slide further out to the front so that the pelvis can remain on the floor.

- Try to breathe into the stiffness, letting the spine drop down bit by bit as you remain there.

- Do not let your shoulders come up around your ears. Keep your neck long.

- Hold the position for one minute, breathing quietly as the spine relaxes.

- To come down, bend the elbows and lie the side of your face on the floor.

- Rest for 15 seconds and then repeat five times, trying to get the front of the pelvis as near as possible to the floor.

As a progression:

FROM THE COBRA TO THE POSE OF THE CHILD

- When the hips fall through to the floor with little residual stiffness, you can move into a see-sawing action back and forth.

- Bend the hips by pulling your tummy in hard and pushing your bottom back towards your heels.

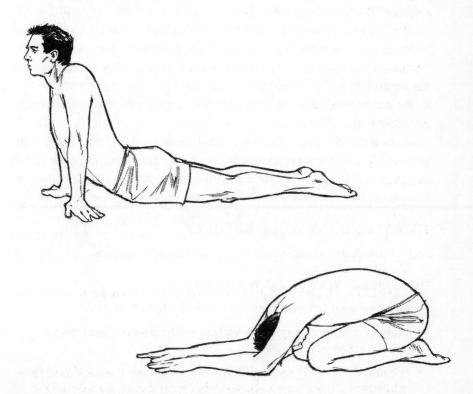

Figure 7.12 The Cobra, progressing to Pose of the Child

- With the top of your feet flat along the floor behind you, nestle your bottom down on your heels.

- Your hands will drag back along the floor a little way; leave them long and relaxed, elbows on the floor.

- Relax the side of your face or your forehead to the floor and remain there for five seconds.

- To rock forwards, slide your hands forward again and after lifting your bottom off your heels, let your hips fall through to the sagging position.

- Count five seconds in this position.

- Repeat nine more times back and forth, counting all the time and trying to let the hips drop more each time.

The Sphinx

A milder version of the Cobra is the Sphinx exercise, where you lie prone, supported on your forearms, as if reading a book on your tummy. Although it does similar things to the Cobra, it is more effective at reversing a very stooped posture. Your back relaxes more in the Sphinx and thoraco-lumbar jamming can be specifically targeted. It is often painful to start with, as the humped middle part of the spine takes a while to drop through and sag. Your tummy and gluteal muscles may clench automatically to prevent the spine letting go but gradually this eases and the spine drops forward the longer you stay there.

Getting out of the Sphinx is often uncomfortable (even for healthy backs) and you may have to rock your hips from left to right, first gently and then with more gusto, before you can lift your hips back from the floor. It may be necessary to roll onto your back and ease your castness by rocking your knees to your chest. This becomes less necessary as your mobility improves. I often manually mobilise stiff thoraco-lumbar spines in the Sphinx position.

THE CORRECT WAY TO DO THE SPHINX

- Lie prone on a carpeted floor with a pillow under your pelvis.

- Push up to support your upper body on both forearms, your elbows directly below your shoulders.

- Let your shoulders relax so your shoulder blades poke out and your spine is free to sag.

- Try to breathe into the stiffness and avoid tensing the spine as it moves through its jammed phase before it drops through to the floor.

- Don't hold onto your spine by tensing the tummy and gluteal muscles. Make them let go so the spine can drop down, one cog at a time.

- Hold the position for one minute and then gently begin to tip your pelvis from left to right in preparation for getting up.

- If you are not too stiff, you can push your bottom back to get up.

- If it hurts too much, roll over onto your back and rock your knees to your chest until the stiffness passes off.

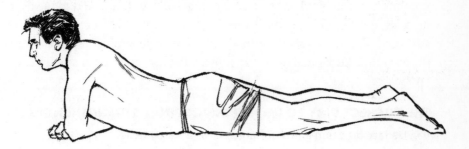

Figure 7.13 The Sphinx

Intrinsics strengthening

This is the ultimate form of spinal strengthening. It is done face down, off the end of a table, with someone holding your feet as you lower your head to the floor and return to horizontal. It is the big brother to the strengthening part of toe touching in the standing position. But because there is a much longer leverage when the spine is suspended out in mid-air off the end of the table, the muscles work much harder to unfurl the spine. The proper action involves a humping movement of the lower back, followed by a wave-like undulation along the spine, with the head coming up last.

This is a very effective way of building up the strength of all the intrinsic muscles of the spine. Longissimus and iliocostalis are strengthened when they make the lumbar vertebrae slide backwards in a reverse gliding action and multifidus is strengthened when it pulls the tails of the vertebrae to slot them back from their tipped forward position.

As well as being the most effective way of strengthening the intrinsics, the horizontal exercise is also the most stable. By contrast, toe touches require more advanced coordination. If you have an unstable segment you never start off from the vertical position, always the horizontal. You may be unlucky enough to get slippage of a vertebra while doing toe touches which will be painful, shake your confidence and leave the problem segment more irritable.

If you want brute strength for a spine which is weak you would go straight to the horizontal form of the intrinsics exercise, doing as many repetitions as your spine can take. But if you want to gradually build up the strength of a very weak, poorly controlled segment, you have to start off doing just a few horizontal intrinsics. These strengthen the segment in its most stable position and then as the control builds up, you progress to the toe touches from a standing position. By then the reaction time will have improved in the deep muscles and the defence mechanisms of the weak segment will be more advanced. When the general level of irritability of the problem segment is on the wane, the horizontal intrinsics provide the higher levels of strength and endurance.

THE CORRECT WAY TO DO INTRINSIC SPINAL STRENGTHENING

- Lie face down on a firm surface such as a sturdy table.

- Place a pillow at the edge of the table and with somebody holding your feet, move up the table so your two hip bones are on the pillow.

- Allow your upper body to drop down towards the floor, putting a hand out to take your weight on the floor.

- Fold your arms across your chest and let your upper body hang down, making an angle of 90° at the hips.

- From this starting position, tighten your buttocks and pull your tummy in, rolling the pelvis back.

- Continuing this very powerful contraction, unfurl along the length of the spine one vertebra at a time, with your head coming up last. Do not attempt to hyperextend beyond the horizontal position.

- To return to the floor, duck the head down and do the movement in reverse.

- At the bottom of the cycle, hang for a moment, completely relaxed, before continuing.

- Repeat ten times.

Figure 7.14 Spinal intrinsics

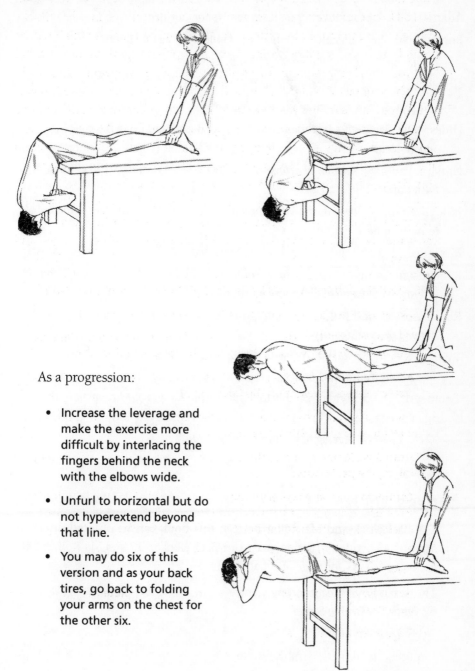

As a progression:

- Increase the leverage and make the exercise more difficult by interlacing the fingers behind the neck with the elbows wide.

- Unfurl to horizontal but do not hyperextend beyond that line.

- You may do six of this version and as your back tires, go back to folding your arms on the chest for the other six.

REFERENCES

Adams, M.A., *Biomechanics of the Lumbar Motion Segment*

Bogduk, Nikolai, *Clinical Anatomy of the Lumbar Spine and Sacrum*

——, *The Innervation of the Intervertebral Discs*

Grieve, G.P., *Common Vertebral Joint Problems*

——, *Referred Pain and other Clinical Features*

Hides, Julie, *Multifidus Inhibition in Acute Low Back Pain: Recovery is not Spontaneous*

Hodges, Paul, *Dysfunction of Transversus Abdominus Associated with Chronic Low Back Pain*

Jull, Gwendolen, *Towards the Validation of a Clinical Test for the Deep Abdominal Muscles in Back Pain Patients*

Macintosh, J. and Bogduk, N., *The Anatomy and Function of the Lumbar Muscles*

Richardson, Carolyn, *Muscle Control in Spinal Instability: Advancement Through Interaction of Clinical Skills and Scientific Research*

Richardson, C. and Jull, G.A., *Concepts of Assessment and Rehabilitation for Active Lumbar Stability*

Taylor, J.R. and Twomey, L.T., *Structure and Function of the Lumbar Zygapophyseal (Facet) Joints*

Twomey, L.T. and Taylor, J.R., *Factors Influencing Ranges of Movement of the Spine*

——, *The Effects of Ageing in the Intervertebral Discs*

ORDERS

The BackBlock and Ma Roller used in this book can be ordered direct by sending a cheque or money order (for BackBlock: $55 and Ma Roller: $40, inclusive of GST, postage and packing) to:

The Sarah Key Physiotherapy Centre
6th Floor, 44 Bridge Street
SYDNEY NSW 2000

Inquiries email: net@SarahKey.com

Index